The Vibrant Anti-Inflammatory Cookbook

Healthy Anti-Inflammatory Recipes For beginners

Thomas Jollif

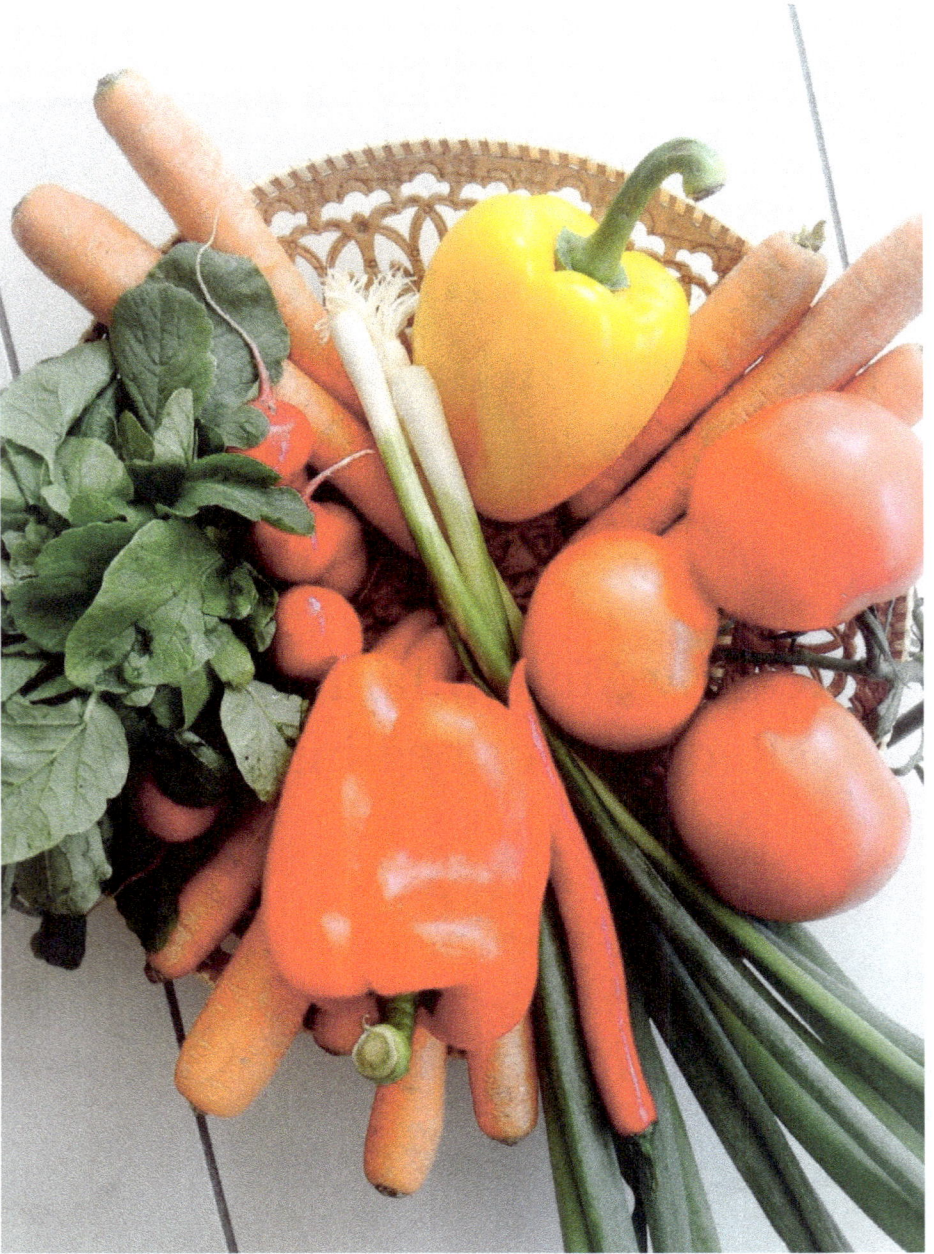

by reading this document, the reader agrees that under no circumstances is the author responsible for any losses, direct or indirect, which are incurred as a result of the use of information contained within this document, including, but not limited to, — errors, omissions, or inaccuracies.

Table of Contents

BREAKFASTS

Oatmeal-Applesauce Muffins

Time To Prepare: fifteen minutes

Time to Cook: twenty-five minutes

Yield: Servings 12

Ingredients:

Topping

- 1 tbsp. brown sugar
- 1 tbsp. unsalted butter, melted
- 1/4 cup rolled oats
- 1/8 tsp. cinnamon

Muffins

- ½ c. brown sugar
- ½ c. unsweetened applesauce
- ½ tsp. Baking soda
- ½ tsp. Cinnamon
- ½ tsp. Salt
- ½ tsp. sugar
- 1 c. nonfat milk
- 1 c. old fashioned rolled oats (not instant)

- 1 c. whole wheat flour
- 1 tsp. Baking powder
- 2 egg whites
- raisins or nuts (opt.)

Directions:

1. To begin, first, presoak the oats in milk for an hour,
2. Set the oven to 400°F then grease a standard 12-cup muffin pan with cooking spray or use paper liners.
3. In a mixing container, mix oat-milk mixture, applesauce, and egg whites. Blend well and save for later.
4. In a different container, put together the whole wheat flour, brown sugar, baking powder, baking soda, salt, sugar, and cinnamon then mix.
5. Slowly put wet ingredients to dry ingredients and blend until just blended, but do not over mix the batter as it will make the muffins firm. Put in raisins or nuts (opt.).
6. Prepare topping: In a small container, whisk together the oats, brown sugar, and cinnamon. Put in in melted butter and toss lightly using a fork to coat ingredients.
7. Fill each muffin cup 2/3 full of batter. Drizzle topping on the top of each batter-filled muffin cup. Tap the pan gently on the counter to even out the batter. Put muffin

pan in preheated oven and cook for twenty to twenty-five minutes or until a toothpick put in the center of one of the muffins comes out clean. Remove from the oven and allow it to sit for five minutes before you serve.

Nutritional Info: Calories: 115 kcal ‖ Protein: 5.06 g ‖ Fat: 2.57 g ‖ Carbohydrates: 22.33 g

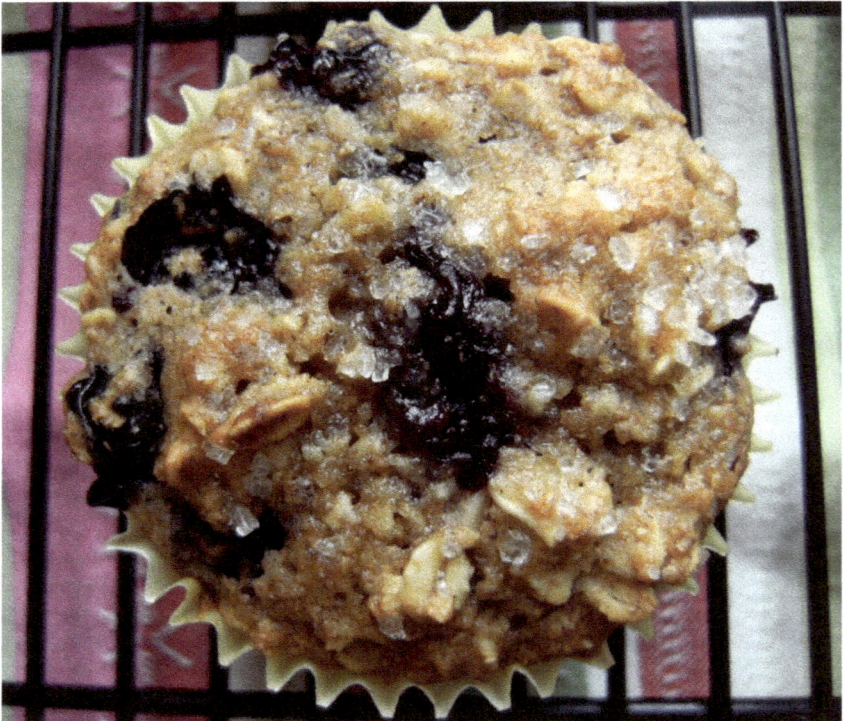

Oatmeal-Raisin Scones

Time To Prepare: ten minutes

Time to Cook: fifteen minutes

Yield: Servings 6

Ingredients:

- ½ cup all-purpose flour
- ½ teaspoon salt
- ½ teaspoon vanilla
- 1 cup raisins
- 1 egg white
- 1½ cups rolled oats
- 11/8teaspoons baking powder
- 2 eggs or ½ cup egg substitute
- 2 tablespoons granulated sugar
- 2 tablespoons wheat germ
- 2/3 cup buttermilk
- 3 tablespoons sugar
- 6 tablespoons cold unsalted butter

Directions:

1. Preheat your oven to 400°F. Coat a baking pan w/ parchment paper or spray lightly with oil. Grind half of the oats into flour in a food processor.

2. Mix remaining oats, oat flour, all-purpose flour, wheat germ, sugar, salt, baking powder, and butter in a food processor using a metal blade. Process until mixture looks like cornmeal.

3. In a huge container, put together eggs, buttermilk, and vanilla then whisk. Mix in raisins using a spatula or wooden spoon.

4. Place the dry ingredients and fold in using a spatula. Drop scones into rounds onto the readied baking sheet.

5. Brush scones with egg white and dust with granulated sugar. Bake for fifteen minutes.

Nutritional Info: Calories: 456 ‖ Fat: 16 g ‖ Protein: 13 g ‖ Sodium: 277 mg ‖ Fiber: 6 g ‖ Carbohydrates: 70 g

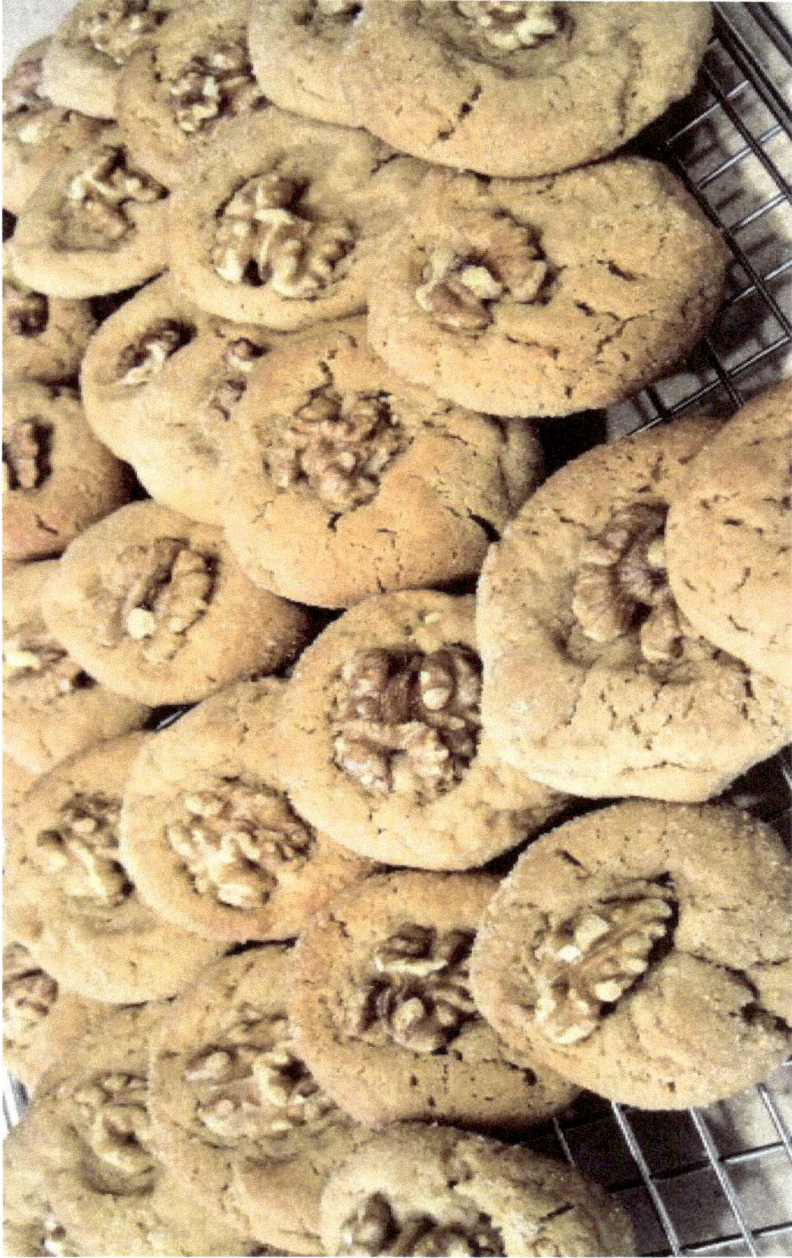

Omega-3-rich Cold Banana Breakfast

Time To Prepare: ten minutes

Time to Cook: 0 minutes

Yield: Servings 2

Ingredients:

- ½ cup cold milk
- 1 big cut Banana
- 2 tbsp. flaxseeds
- 2 tbsp. ground coconut
- 4 tbsp. sesame seeds
- 4 tbsp. sunflower seeds

Directions:

1. Combine the milk and honey on your breakfast container. Use your coffee grinder to grind all the seeds.
2. Put in the ground seeds to the honey and milk mixture. Put the cut bananas neatly on top. Drizzle the ground coconuts for added flavor.

Nutritional Info: Calories: 393 kcal ‖ Protein: 14.85 g ‖ Fat: 27.63 g ‖ Carbohydrates: 27.37 g

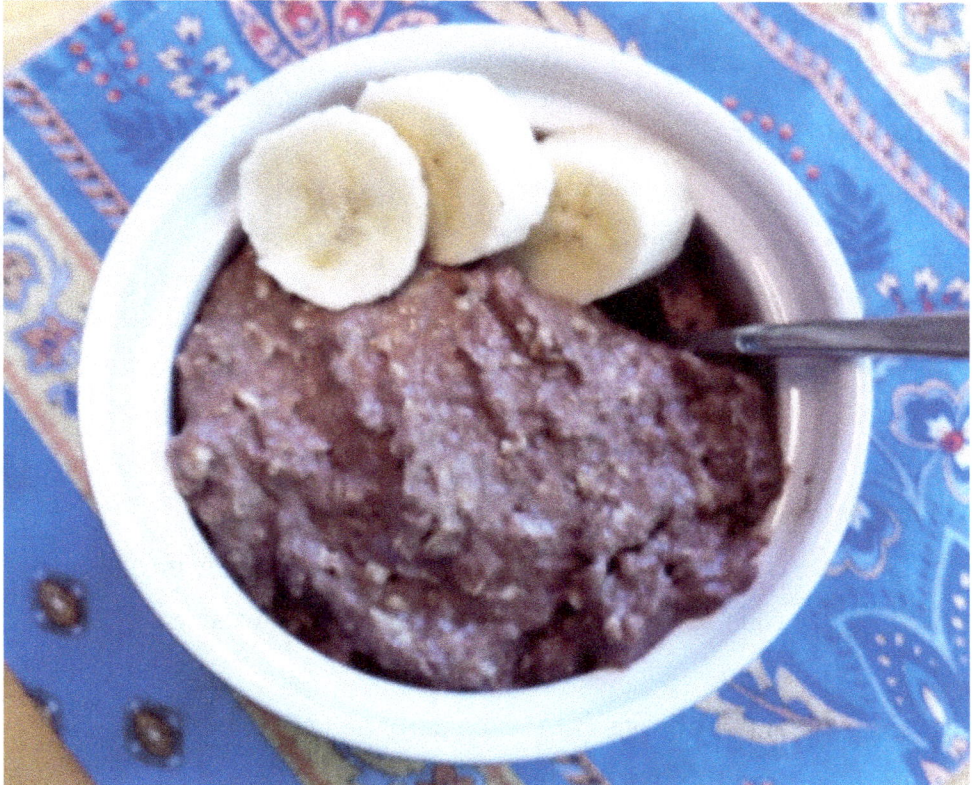

Oven-Poached Eggs

Time To Prepare: 2minutes

Time to Cook: 11minutes

Yield: Servings 4

Ingredients:

- 2 cups of ice cubes
- 2 cups water, chilled
- 6 eggs, at room temperature
- Ice bath
- Water

Directions:

1. Set the oven to 350°F. Put 2 cups of water into a deep roasting tin, and place it into the lowest rack of the oven.

2. Put one egg into each cup of cupcake/muffin tins, together with one tablespoon of water.

3. Cautiously place muffin tins into the middle rack of the oven.

4. Bake eggs for about forty-five minutes.

5. Remove the heat instantly. Take off the muffin tins from the oven and set on a cake rack to cool before extracting eggs.

6. Pour ice bath ingredients into a big heat-resistant container.

7. Bring the eggs into an ice bath to stop the cooking process. After ten minutes, drain eggs well. Use as required.

Nutritional Info: Calories: 357 kcal ‖ Protein: 17.14 g ‖ Fat: 24.36 g ‖ Carbohydrates: 16.19 g

Peaches with Honey Almond Ricotta

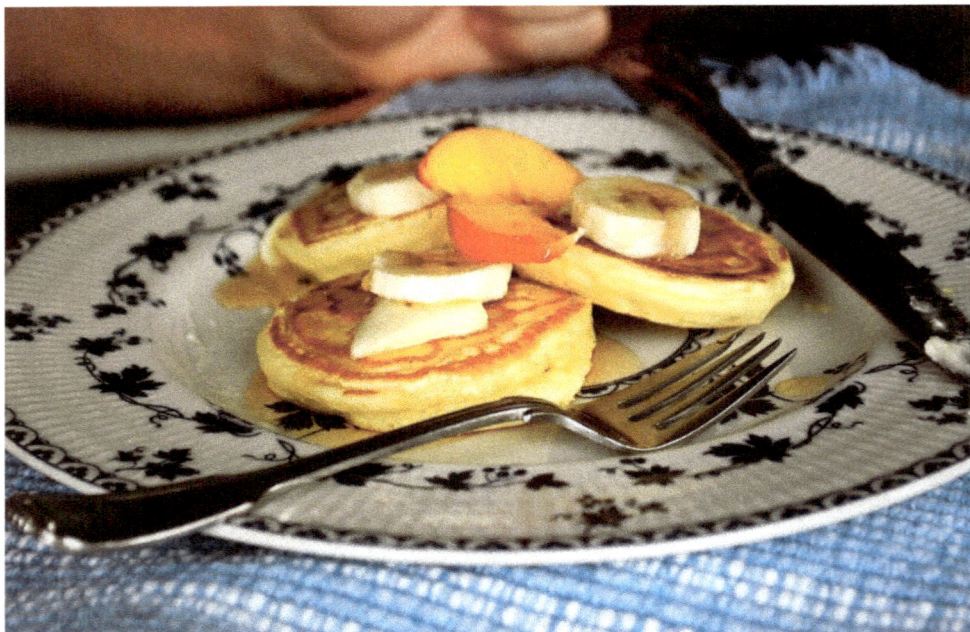

Time To Prepare: fifteen minutes

Time to Cook: 0 minutes

Yield: Servings 4-6

Ingredients:

- ¼ cup Almond extract
- ¼ cup Peaches, cut

- ½ cup Almonds, thin slices
- 1 cup Ricotta, skim milk
- 1 tsp. Honey
- Bread, whole grain bagel or toast
- Spread
- To Serve

Directions:

1. Combine the almond extract, honey, ricotta, and almonds.
2. Spread one tablespoon of this mix on toasted bread and cover with peaches.

Nutritional Info: Calories 230 ‖ 9 grams Protein ‖ 8g Fat ‖ 37g carbs ‖ 3 g fiber ‖ 34g sugar

Peanut Butter-Banana Muffins

Time To Prepare: fifteen minutes

Time to Cook: twenty-five minutes

Yield: Servings 12

Ingredients:

- ½ tsp. Baking soda
- ½ tsp. salt
- ¾ c. light brown sugar
- 1 c. low-fat buttermilk
- 1 c. mashed banana (about 3 bananas)
- 1 c. old-fashioned oats
- 1 tsp. Baking powder
- 1½ c. all-purpose flour
- 2 big eggs
- 2 tbsp. Applesauce
- 6 tbsp. creamy peanut butter

Directions:

1. Bring a small nonstick frying pan on moderate heat and spray lightly with cooking spray. Put in in the bell pepper and onion and sauté for one to two minutes, or until both are soft and the onion translucent.

2. In a small container, crack in eggs and whisk. Put in in milk; whisk until well-mixed. Pour eggs into the pan and cook, regularly stirring until eggs are scrambled to your preference.
3. To serve, spoon half the egg mixture into each tortilla, wrap, before you serve. Try serving with a side of fresh fruit for a complete meal.

Nutritional Info: Calories: 187 kcal ‖ Protein: 8.12 g ‖ Fat: 6.25 g ‖ Carbohydrates: 27.82 g

Poached Salmon Egg Toast

Time To Prepare: ten minutes

Time to Cook: 4 minutes

Yield: Servings 2

Ingredients:

- ¼ tsp. Black pepper
- ¼ tsp. Lemon juice
- 1 tbsp. Scallions, cut thin
- 1/8 tsp. Salt
- 2 Eggs, poached
- 2 tbs. Avocado, mashed
- 4 oz. Salmon, smoked
- Bread, two slices rye or whole-grain toasted

Directions:

1. Put in lemon juice to avocado with pepper and salt. Spread the mixed avocado over the toasted bread slices.
2. Lay smoked salmon over toast and top with a poached egg. Top with cut scallions.

Nutritional Info: Calories 389 ‖ 17.2 grams Fat ‖ 33.5 grams Protein ‖ 31.5 grams carbs ‖ 1.3 grams sugar ‖ 9.3 grams fiber ‖

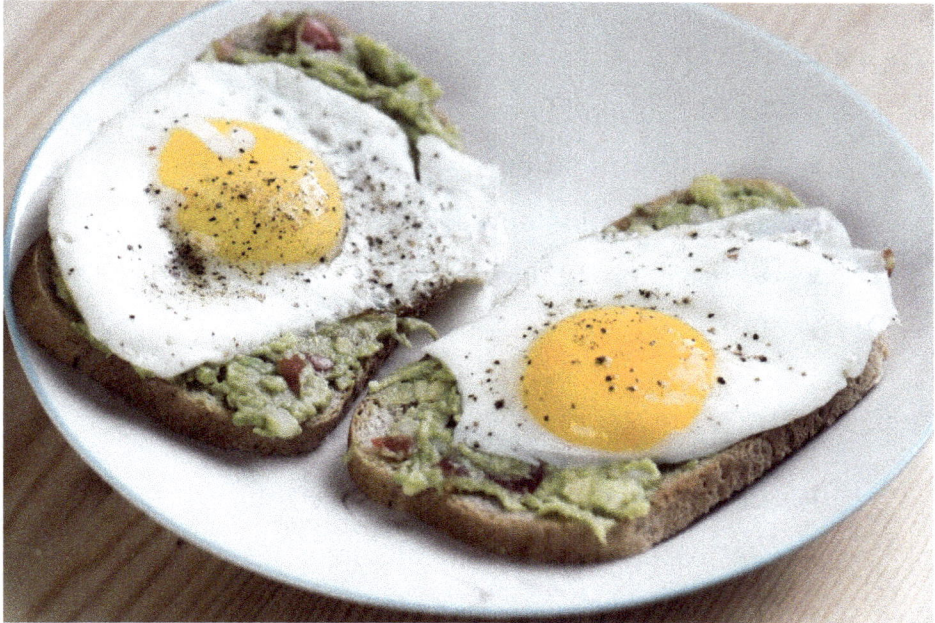

Pumpkin & Banana Waffles

Time To Prepare: fifteen minutes

Time to Cook: five minutes

Yield: Servings 4

Ingredients:

- ½ cup almond flour
- ½ cup coconut flour
- ½ cup pumpkin puree
- ½ teaspoon ground cloves
- ½ teaspoon ground nutmeg
- ¾ cup almond milk
- ¾ teaspoon ground ginger
- 1 tsp baking soda
- 1½ teaspoons ground cinnamon
- 2 medium bananas, peeled and cut
- 2 tablespoons olive oil
- 5 big organic eggs
- Salt, to taste

Directions:

1. Preheat the waffle iron, and after that, grease it.

2. In a sizable container, combine flours, baking soda, and spices.
3. In a blender, put the rest of the ingredients and pulse till smooth.
4. Put in flour mixture and pulse till
5. In preheated waffle iron, put in the required quantity of mixture.
6. Cook roughly 4-5 minutes.
7. Repeat using the rest of the mixture.

Nutritional Info: Calories: 357.2 ‖ Fat: 28.5g ‖ Carbohydrates: 19.7g ‖ Fiber: 4g ‖ Protein: 14g

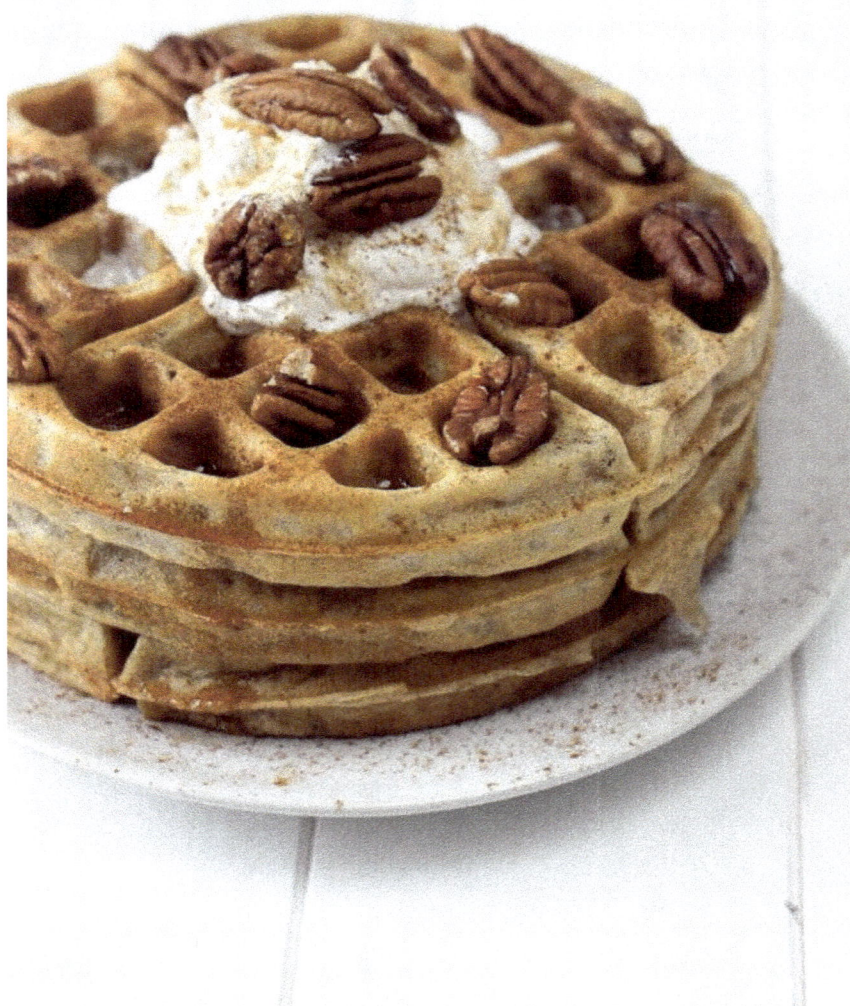

Pumpkin Pancakes

Time To Prepare: twenty-five minutes

Time to Cook: ten minutes

Yield: Servings 6

Ingredients:

- ½ cup pumpkin puree
- 1 cup coconut cream
- 1 ounce egg white Protein
- 1 tablespoon chai masala
- 1 tablespoon swerve
- 1 teaspoon baking powder
- 1 teaspoon coconut oil
- 1 teaspoon vanilla extract
- 2 ounces flax seeds; ground
- 2 ounces hazelnut flour
- 3 eggs
- 5 drops stevia

Directions:

1. In a container, mix flax seeds with hazelnut flour, egg white Protein baking powder and chai masala and stir.

2. In another container, mix coconut cream with vanilla extract, pumpkin puree, eggs, stevia, and swerve and stir thoroughly.

3. Mix the 2 mixtures and stir thoroughly.

4. Heat a pan with the oil on moderate to high heat; pour 1/6 of the batter, spread into a circle, cover, decrease the heat to low, cook for about three minutes on each side and move to a plate

5. Repeat the process using the rest of the mixture and serve pumpkin pancakes immediately.

Nutritional Info: Calories: 400 ‖ Fat: 23 ‖ Fiber: 4 ‖ Carbohydrates: 5 ‖ Protein: 21

Quinoa & Beans Burgers

Time To Prepare: fifteen minutes
Time to Cook: 55 minutes
Yield: Servings 12

Ingredients:

- ½ cup dry quinoa
- ½ cup fresh cilantro, chopped
- ½ teaspoon fresh ginger, grated finely
- ½ teaspoon ground turmeric
- 1 (fifteen oz.) can black beans, drained
- 1 cup cooked corn kernels
- 1 small boiled potato, peeled
- 1 small onion, chopped
- 1 teaspoon chili flakes
- 1 teaspoon flax meal
- 1 teaspoon garlic, minced
- 1 teaspoon ground cumin
- 1 teaspoon paprika
- 1½ cups water
- Freshly ground black pepper, to taste
- Salt, to taste

Directions:

1. In a pan, put in water and quinoa on high heat and provide to its boiling point.
2. Reduce the heat to moderate and simmer for around fifteen-twenty or so minutes.
3. Drain surplus water.
4. Set the oven to 375°F. Coat a sizable baking sheet that has a parchment paper.
5. In a sizable container, put in quinoa and rest of the ingredients.
6. Use a fork to mix till well blended.
7. Make equal-sized patties from the mixture.
8. Position the patties onto the readied baking sheet in the single layer.
9. Bake for around 20-twenty-five minutes.
10. Cautiously, alter the side and cook for approximately 8-ten minutes.

Nutritional Info: Calories: 400 ‖ Fat: 9g ‖ Carbohydrates: 27g ‖ Fiber: 12g ‖ Protein: 38g

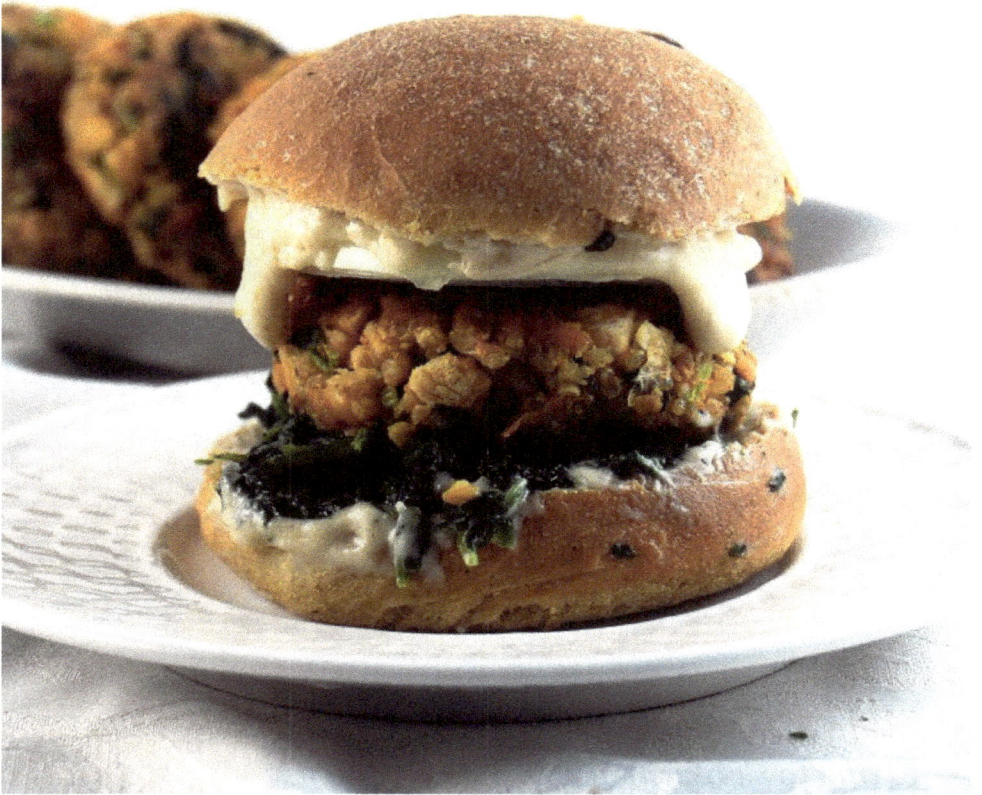

SMOOTHIES AND DRINKS

Peachy Keen Smoothie

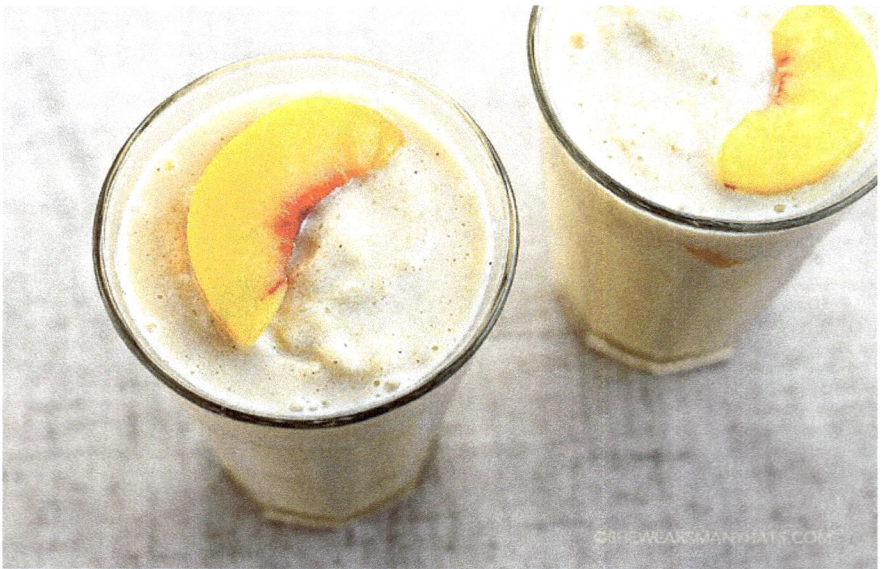

Time To Prepare: five minutes

Time to Cook: 0 minutes

Yield: Servings 2

Ingredients:

- 1 ½ cups of frozen peaches
- 1 cup of almond milk

- 1 small frozen banana
- 2 tbsp. of raw hemp seeds
- 6 to 8 ice cubes
- Pinch of ground ginger

Directions:

1. Mix the smoothie ingredients in your high-speed blender.
2. Pulse the ingredients a few times to cut them up.
3. Combine the mixture on the highest speed setting for thirty to 60 seconds.
4. Pour into glasses and serve.

Nutritional Info: Calories: 388 kcal ‖ Protein: 10.59 g ‖ Fat: 11.93 g ‖ Carbohydrates: 64.08 g

Pineapple & Ginger Juice

Time To Prepare: five minutes

Time to Cook: 0 minutes

Yield: Servings 2

Ingredients:

- 2 apples, cored, chopped
- 2 cucumbers, chopped
- 2 cups chopped pineapple
- 2 cups spinach
- 2 inches ginger, peeled, cut
- 2 lemons, peeled, halved
- 8 celery stalks, chopped

Directions:

1. Juice together all the ingredients in a juicer.
2. Pour into 2 glasses before you serve.

Nutritional Info: Calories: 339 kcal ‖ Protein: 7.44 g ‖ Fat: 4.23 g ‖ Carbohydrates: 75.38 g

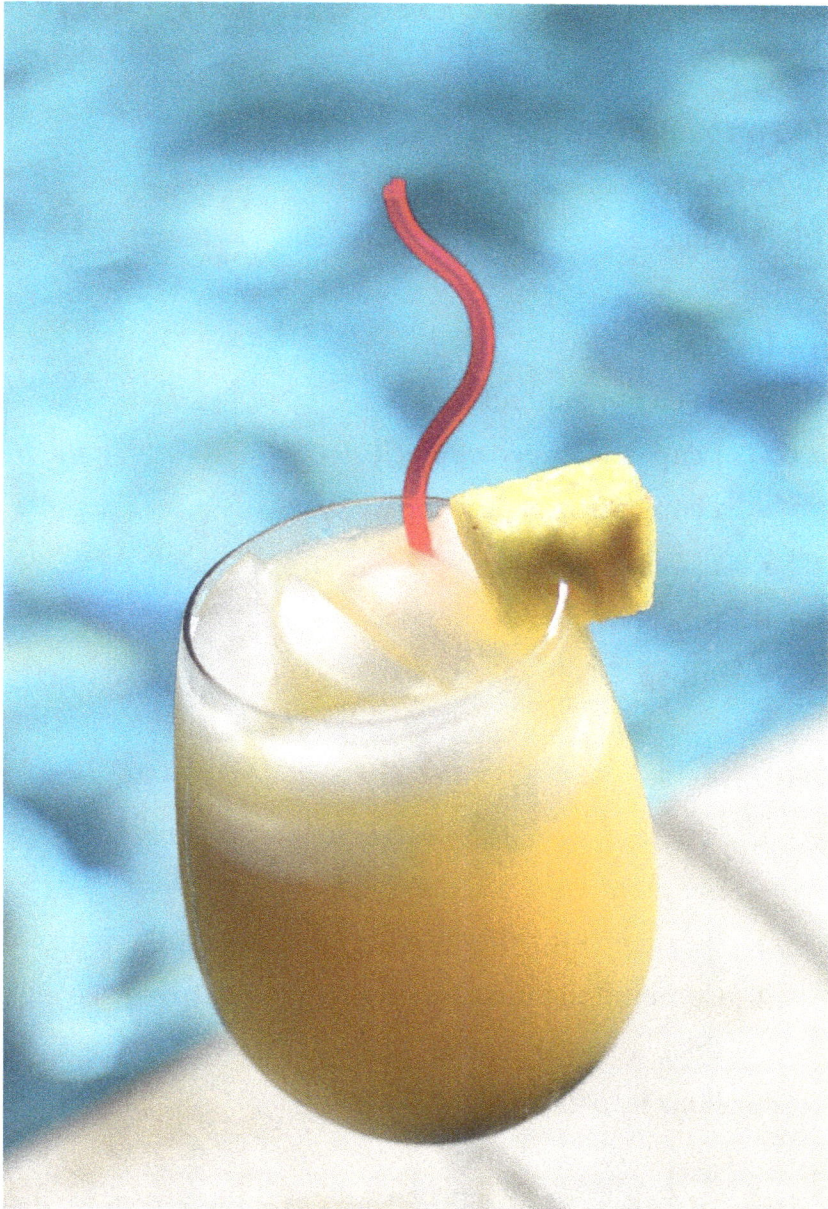

Pineapple and Greens Smoothie

Time To Prepare: five minutes

Time to Cook: 0 minutes

Yield: Servings 2

Ingredients:

- ¾ cup of almond milk
- 1 cup of chopped spinach
- 1 cup of frozen pineapple
- 1 small frozen banana
- 1 tbsp. of honey
- 2 tbsp. Of chia seeds

Directions:

1. Mix the smoothie ingredients in your high-speed blender.
2. Pulse the ingredients a few times to cut them up.
3. Combine the mixture on the highest speed setting for thirty to 60 seconds.
4. Pour into glasses and serve.

Nutritional Info: Calories: 272 kcal ‖ Protein: 5.27 g ‖ Fat: 4.5 g ‖ Carbohydrates: 56.37 g

Pineapple- Ginger Smoothie

Time To Prepare: five minutes

Time to Cook: 0 minutes

Yield: Servings 1

Ingredients:

- ½ inch thick ginger, cut
- 1 cup coconut milk
- 1 cup pineapple slice

Directions:

1. Put all ingredients in a blender.
2. Pulse until the desired smoothness is achieved.
3. Chill before you serve.

Nutritional Info: Calories 299 ‖ Fat: 8 g ‖ Protein: 9 g ‖ Carbohydrates: 51 g

Pineapple Smoothie

Time To Prepare: ten minutes

Time to Cook: 0 minutes

Yield: Servings 2

Ingredients:

- 1 1/2 cups pineapple chunks
- 1 cup coconut water
- 1 orange, peeled and slice into quarters
- 1 tbsp. fresh grated ginger
- 1 tsp. chia seeds
- 1 tsp. turmeric powder
- A pinch black pepper

Directions:

1. In your blender, combine the coconut water with the orange, pineapple, ginger, chia seeds, turmeric, and black pepper.
2. Pulse thoroughly, pour into a glass.

Makes for a great breakfast!

Nutritional Info: Calories: 151 ‖ Fat: 2 g ‖ Protein: 4 g ‖ Carbohydrates: 12 g ‖ Fiber: 6 g

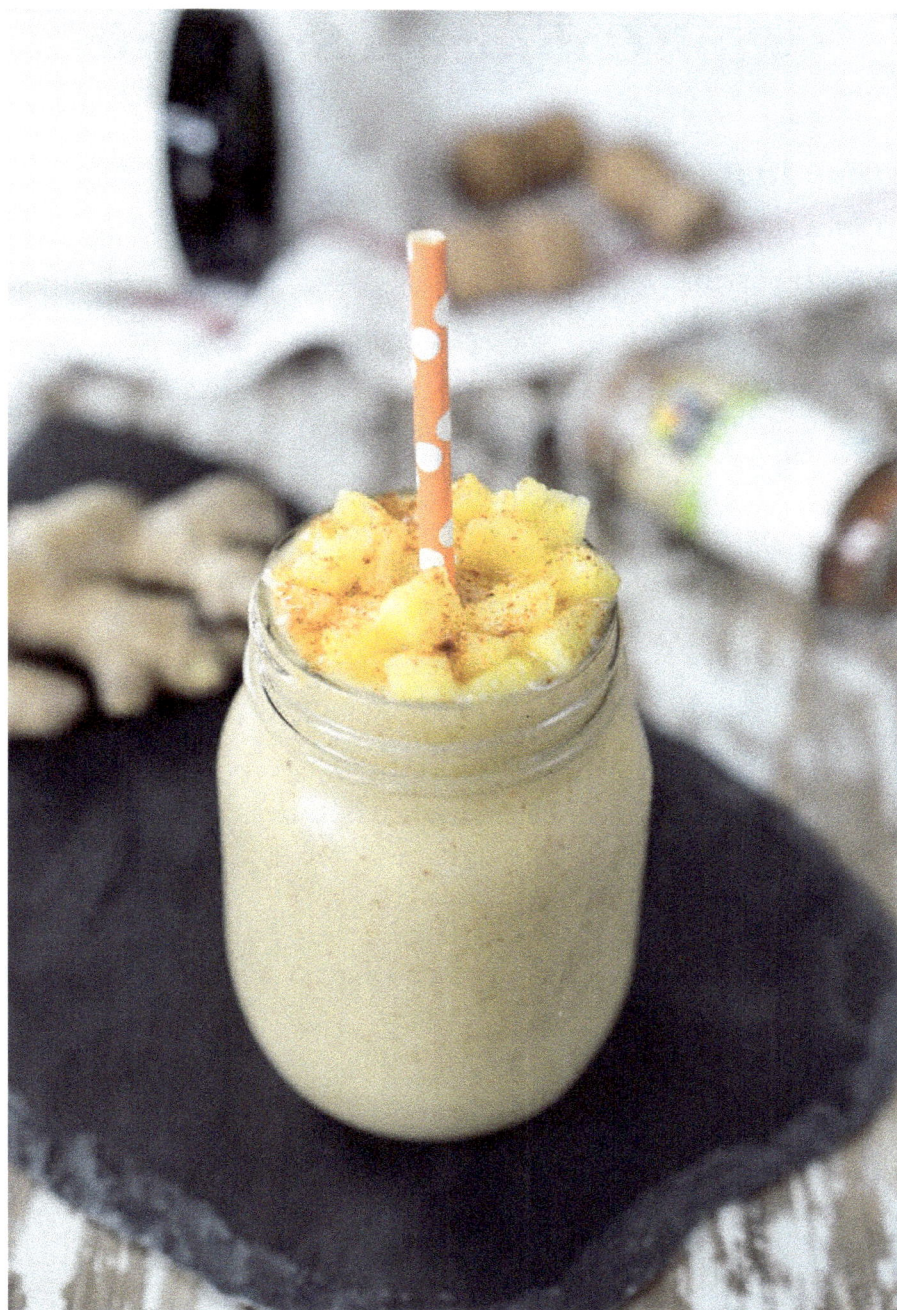

Pink California Smoothie

Time To Prepare: ten minutes

Time to Cook: 0 minutes

Yield: Servings 1

Ingredients:

- 1 container (8 oz.) lemon yogurt
- 1/3 cup orange juice
- 7 big strawberries

Directions:

1. Put in everything to a blender jug.
2. Cover the jug firmly.
3. Blend until the desired smoothness is achieved. Serve and enjoy!

Nutritional Info: Calories: 144 ‖ Fat: 0.4 g ‖ Protein: 5.6 g ‖ Carbohydrates: 8 g ‖ Fiber: 2.3 g

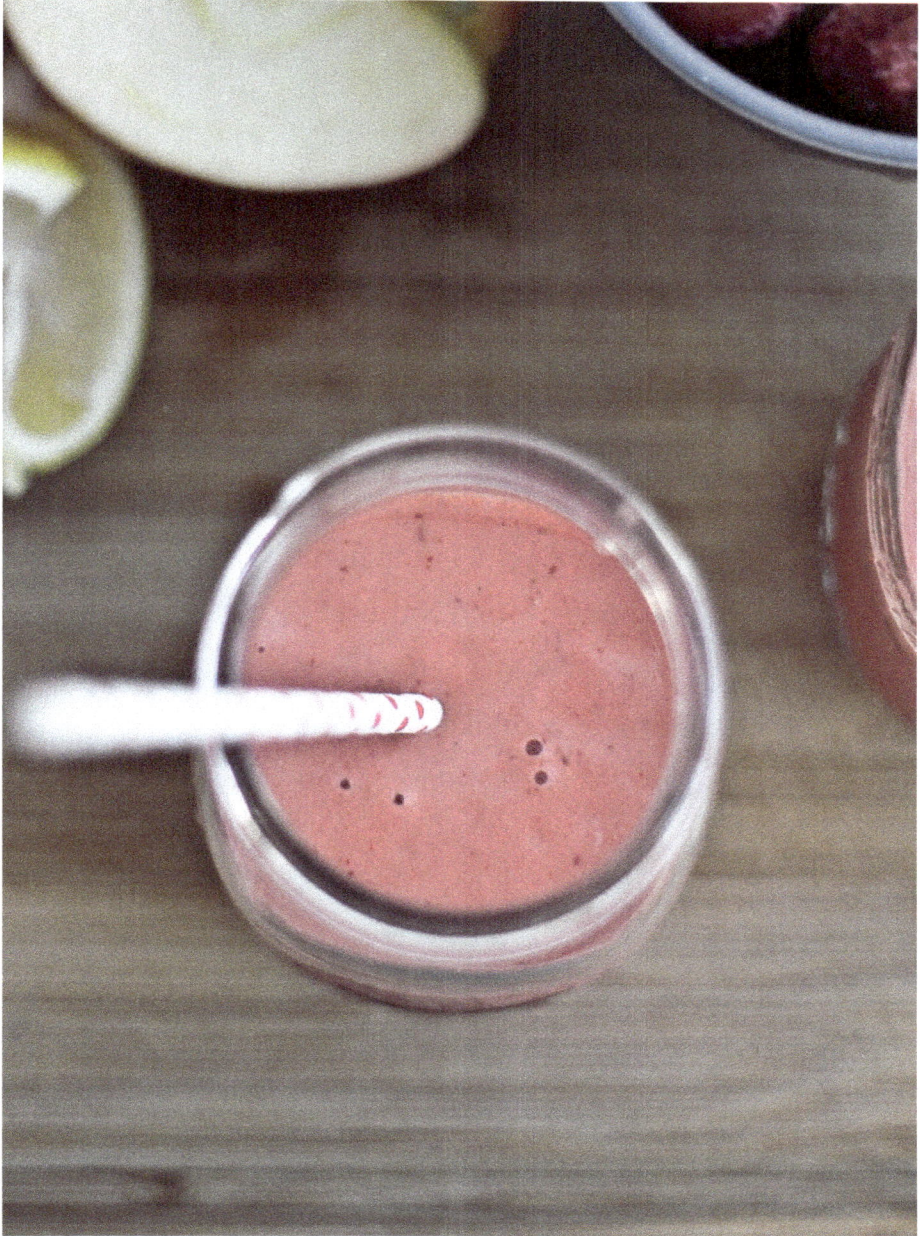

Pumpkin Pie Smoothie

Time To Prepare: five minutes

Time to Cook: 0 minutes

Yield: Servings 2

Ingredients:

- ½ Cup Pumpkin, Canned & Unsweetened
- 1 Banana
- 1 Cup Almond Milk
- 1 Teaspoon Ground Cinnamon
- 1 Teaspoon Ground Nutmeg
- 1 Teaspoon Maple Syrup, Pure
- 1 Teaspoon Vanilla Extract Pure
- 2 Tablespoons Almond Butter, Heaping
- 2-3 Ice Cubes

Directions:

Blend all ingredients together until the desired smoothness is achieved.

Nutritional Info: Calories: 235 ‖ Protein: 5.6 Grams ‖ Fat: 11 Grams ‖ Carbohydrates: 27.8 Grams

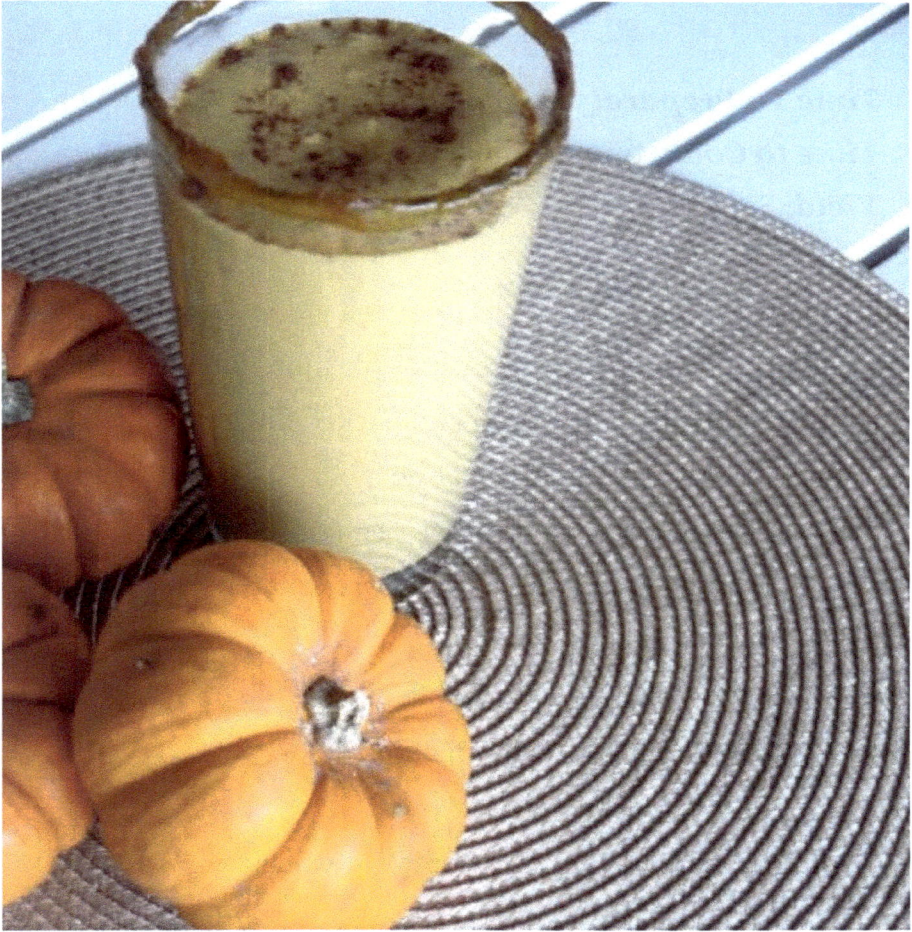

SIDES

Rice with Pistachios

Time To Prepare: ten minutes
Time to Cook: twenty minutes
Yield: Servings 6

Ingredients:

- ¼ cup of raw pistachios (or more for decoration)
- ½ cup of chopped and packed dill leaves
- ½ teaspoon of turmeric
- 1 ½ cups of Basmati rice (rinsed in a colander and soaked in water for approximately 30 minutes, or more)
- 1 teaspoon of vegetable oil
- 1 thinly cut medium onion
- 2 dry baby leaves
- 3 cups of vegetable stock or water
- 5 pods of slightly crushed green cardamom
- Ground black pepper (to taste)
- Salt, to taste

Directions:

1. In a big deep cooking pan, warm the oil and put in the cardamom. Heat it for approximately 1 minute until it turns smildly brown and put in the onion. Sauté for approximately 1-2 minutes.

2. Mix in the dill leaves, turmeric and pistachios. Then put in the rice and stir-fry for approximately one minute.

3. Combine the vegetable stock, black pepper and salt to taste, stir it well and bring it to its boiling point.

4. Cover the pan using lid and cook on moderate to low heat for approximately fifteen minutes.

5. Take it off from the heat then set aside the rice (covered) for approximately ten minutes. Then fluff it using a fork and put in more pistachios as decorate, if you desire.

6. Enjoy!

Nutritional Info: ‖ Calories: 90 kcal ‖ Protein: 3.36 g ‖ Fat: 5.08 g ‖ Carbohydrates: 8.39 g

Roasted Carrots

Time To Prepare: ten minutes

Time to Cook: forty minutes

Yield: Servings 4

Ingredients:

- ¼ teaspoon ground pepper
- ½ teaspoon rosemary, chopped
- ½ teaspoon salt
- 1 onion, peeled & cut
- 1 teaspoon thyme, chopped
- 2 tablespoons of extra-virgin olive oil
- 8 carrots, peeled & cut

Directions:

1. Preheat the oven to 425 degrees F.
2. Combine the onions and carrots by tossing in a container with rosemary, thyme, pepper, and salt. Spread on your baking sheet.
3. Roast for forty minutes. The onions and carrots must be browning and soft.

Nutritional Info: Calories 126 ‖ Carbohydrates: 16g ‖ Total Fat: 6g ‖ Protein: 2g ‖ Fiber: 4g ‖ Sugar: 8g ‖ Sodium: 286mg

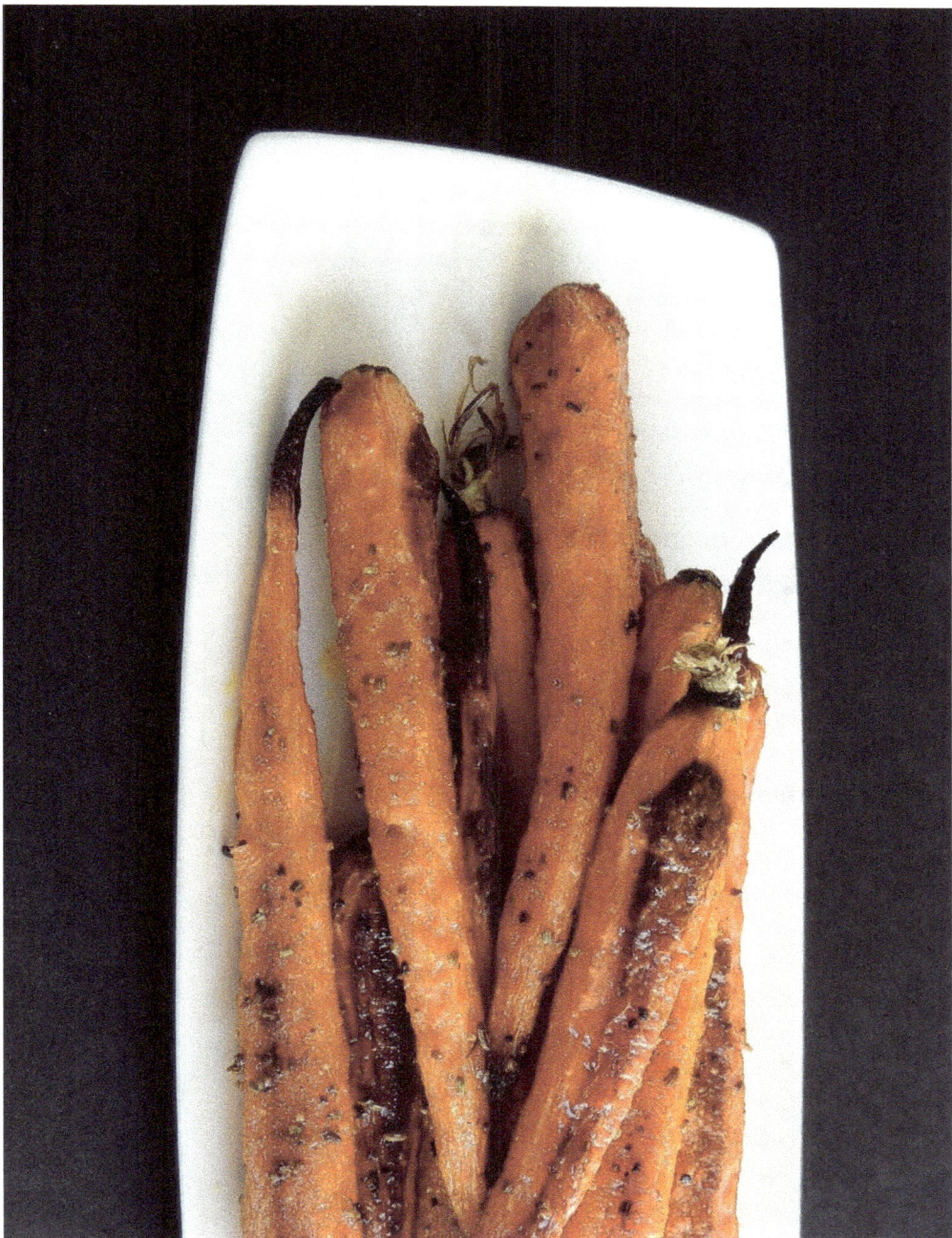

Roasted Curried Cauliflower

Time To Prepare: five minutes

Time to Cook: thirty minutes

Yield: Servings 4

Ingredients:

- ¾ teaspoon salt
- 1 and ½ tablespoon olive oil
- 1 big head cauliflower, cut into florets
- 1 teaspoon cumin seeds
- 1 teaspoon curry powder
- 1 teaspoon mustard seeds

Directions:

1. Preheat the oven to 375 degrees F
2. Grease a baking sheet with cooking spray
3. Take a container and place all ingredients
4. Toss to coat well
5. Position the vegetable on a baking sheet
6. Roast for thirty minutes
7. Serve and enjoy!

Nutritional Info: ‖ Calories: 67 ‖ Fat: 6g ‖ Carbohydrates: 4g ‖ Protein: 2g

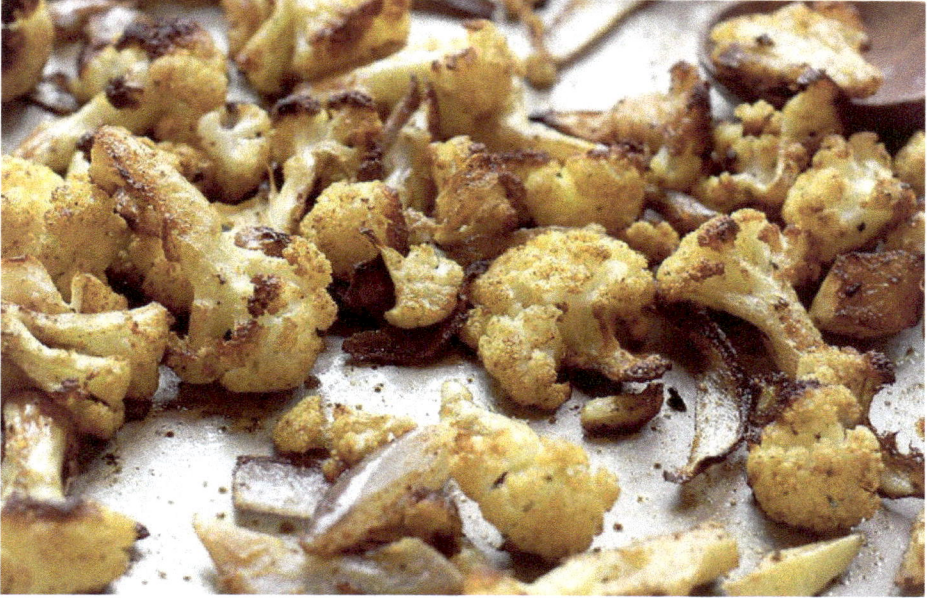

Roasted Parsnips

Time To Prepare: five minutes

Time to Cook: thirty minutes

Yield: Servings 4

Ingredients:

- 1 tablespoon of extra-virgin olive oil
- 1 teaspoon of kosher salt
- 1½ teaspoon of Italian seasoning
- 2 lbs. parsnips
- Chopped parsley for decoration

Directions:

1. Preheat the oven to 400 degrees F.
2. Peel the parsnips. Cut them into one-inch chunks.
3. Now toss with the seasoning, salt, and oil in a container.
4. Spread this on your baking sheet. It must be in a single layer.
5. Roast for half an hour Stir every ten minutes.
6. Move to a plate. Decorate using parsley.

Nutritional Info: Calories 124 ‖ Carbohydrates: 20g ‖ Total Fat: 4g ‖ Protein: 2g ‖ Fiber: 4g ‖ Sugar: 5g ‖ Sodium: 550mg

SAUCES AND DRESSINGS

Homemade Lemon Vinaigrette

Time To Prepare: ten minutes
Time to Cook: 0 minutes
Yield: Servings 2-4

Ingredients:

- ¼ tsp of sea salt
- ½ tsp of Dijon mustard, without preservatives
- ½ tsp of lemon zest
- 1 tsp of honey or maple syrup
- 2 tbsp. of freshly squeezed lemon juice
- 3 tbsp. of extra-virgin olive oil
- Freshly ground black pepper

Directions:

1. Whisk all together the ingredients apart from olive oil and black pepper in a small container. Then progressively put in 3 tbsp. of olive oil while continuously whisking until well blended. Put in some ground black pepper to taste.

2. Put mason jar and place in your fridge for maximum 3 days.
3. Serve with a garden salads.

Nutritional Info: ‖ Calories: 68 kcal ‖ Protein: 1.69 g ‖ Fat: 6.06 g ‖ Carbohydrates: 1.71 g

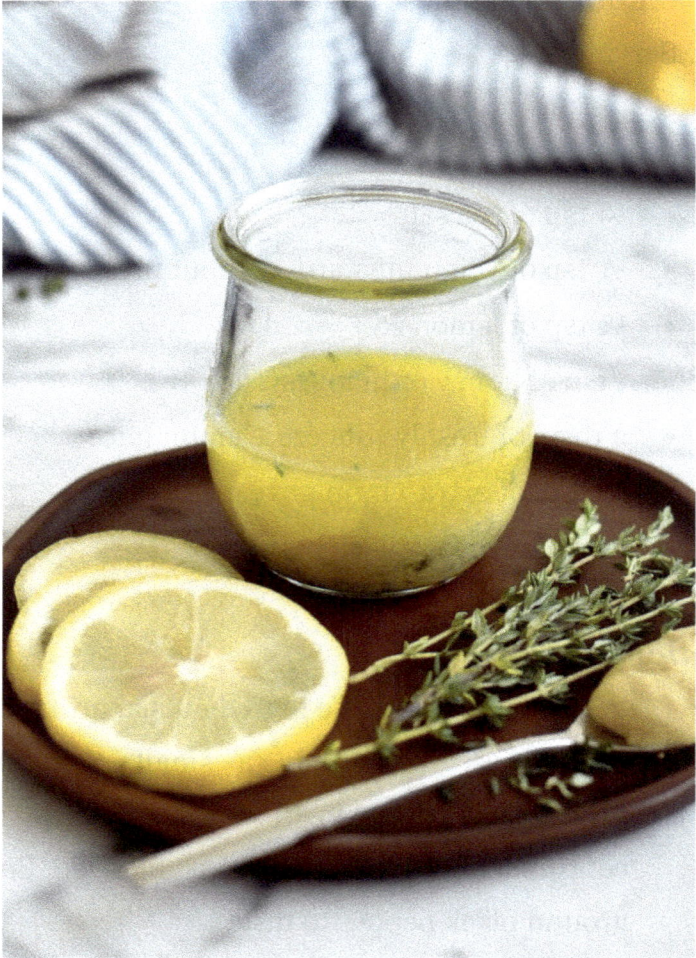

Homemade Ranch

Time To Prepare: ten minutes

Time to Cook: 0 minutes

Yield: Servings 2-4

Ingredients:

- ¼ cup of Greek yogurt
- ¼ tsp Kosher salt
- ½ cup of natural mayonnaise, without preservatives
- ½ tsp of dried dill
- ½ tsp of dried parsley
- ½ tsp of garlic powder
- ½ tsp of onion powder
- ¾ cup of non-dairy milk
- 1/8 tsp Freshly ground black pepper
- 2 tsp of dried chives

Directions:

1. Combine all ingredients apart from the milk into a medium container. Mix together until well blended.
2. Put in in the milk and mix thoroughly.
3. Pour in a mason jar or an airtight container. Serve instantly or place in your fridge for maximum 2 hours

to keep the freshness. Put in your refrigerator for maximum 5 days.

4. Serve with a garden or fruit salad.

Nutritional Info: ‖ Calories: 482 kcal ‖ Protein: 3.55 g ‖ Fat: 51.98 g ‖ Carbohydrates: 1.63 g

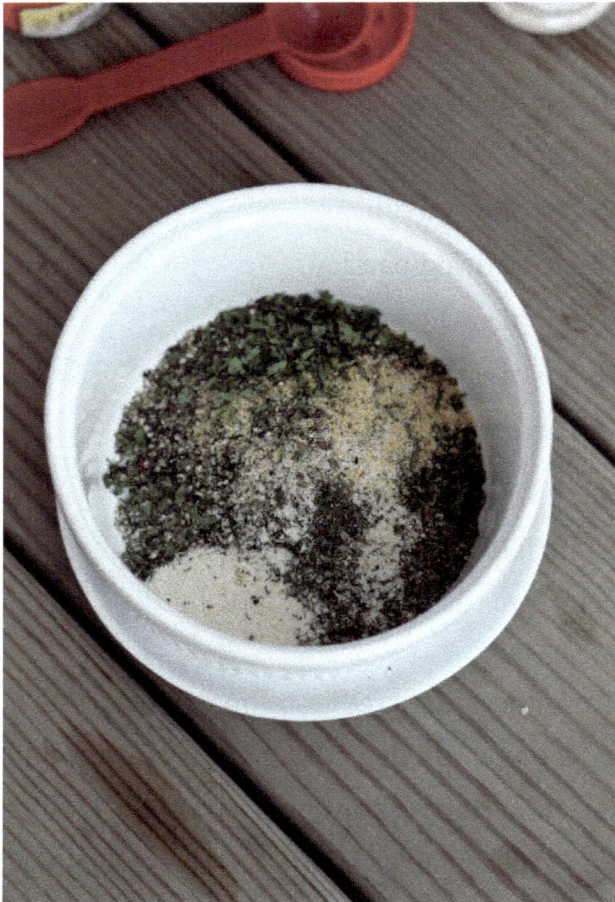

SNACKS

Hummus with Celery

Time To Prepare: fifteen minutes

Time to Cook: 0 minutes

Yield: Servings 4

Ingredients:

- 3 cloves of garlic, crushed
- 2 tablespoons extra virgin olive oil
- ½ teaspoon salt
- ½ teaspoon cumin
- 1 (fifteen–ounce) can chickpeas
- two to three tablespoons water
- Dash of paprika
- 6 stalks celery, cut into two-inch pieces
- 3 tablespoons salsa
- 1/4 cup lemon juice
- 1/4 cup tahini

Directions:

1. Using a food processor mix the lemon juice and tahini for approximately one minute, until it is smooth. Scrape the sides down and process for 30 more seconds.

2. Put in the garlic, olive oil, salt, and cumin. Blend for approximately one minute.

3. Drain the chickpeas, put the half of them on the food processor, and blend for one more minute. Scrape down the sides, put in the other half of the chickpeas, and pulse until smooth, approximately 2 minutes. If it like a little too thick, put in water, 1 tablespoon at a time until you reach the desired consistency.

4. Fill the celery sticks with hummus and drizzle paprika on top.

5. Serve with salsa for dipping.

Nutritional Info: ‖ Calories: 240 kcal ‖ Protein: 9.27 g ‖ Fat: 14.51 g ‖ Carbohydrates: 21.01 g

Kale Chips

Time To Prepare: ten minutes

Time to Cook: 2 hours

Yield: Servings 8

Ingredients:

- ½ teaspoon sea salt
- 1 cup cashews, soaked and softened in water about 2 hours
- 1 cup grated sweet potato
- 2 bunches of curly kale with stems removed, washed and torn into bite-sized pieces
- 2 tablespoons honey
- 2 tablespoons nutritional yeast (found at health food stores)
- 2 tablespoons water
- The juice of 1 lemon

Directions:

1. Place the kale in a huge container and save for later.
2. In a blender or food processor, process the sweet potato, softened cashews yeast, lemon juice, honey, salt, and water until the desired smoothness is

achieved. Place the mixture on the kale and toss with your hands to coat the leaves.

3. Spread the kale leaves out on a big cookie sheet in a single cover without touching.

4. Set the oven to its lowest setting.

5. Prop the oven door slightly ajar and dehydrate the chips for approximately 2 hours flipping the cookie sheet and watching to ensure the chips do not burn.

6. When crunchy, take it out of the oven and allow to cool. Store in an airtight container.

Nutritional Info: ‖ Calories: 40 kcal ‖ Protein: 2.19 g ‖ Fat: 0.87 g ‖ Carbohydrates: 6.39 g

Lemony Ginger Cookies

Time To Prepare: fifteen minutes + thirty minutes chill time

Time to Cook: 10-twelve minutes

Yield: Servings 25

Ingredients:

- ½ cup arrowroot flour
- ½ teaspoon baking soda
- 1 ½ cup coconut butter, softened
- 1 ½ cups stevia
- 1 teaspoon nutritional yeast
- 2 teaspoons vanilla
- 3 inches of ginger root, peeled and diced
- 3/4 teaspoon salt
- Zest of 1 lemon

Directions:

1. Set the oven to 350F, then line two or three cookie sheets using parchment paper.
2. Combine the arrowroot flour, stevia, salt, soda, and yeast in a container.
3. In another container, put the rest of the ingredients and mix thoroughly.

4. Put in the dry ingredients progressively until well blended. If the dough is too soft, put an additional one to 2 tablespoons of arrowroot powder. The dough will stiffen when chilled, so be careful.

5. Cover the dough in parchment and push it flat. Chill for half an hour

6. Take a chunk of the chilled dough and flatten it between two pieces of parchment until it is 1/8 inch thick. Sprinkle with a little arrowroot powder and slice into shapes.

7. Put on baking sheets approximately 1 inch apart and bake ten to twelve minutes. Cool on cookie sheets for fifteen minutes before removing.

Nutritional Info: ‖ Calories: 112 kcal ‖ Protein: 0.44 g ‖ Fat: 11.3 g ‖ Carbohydrates: 2.49 g

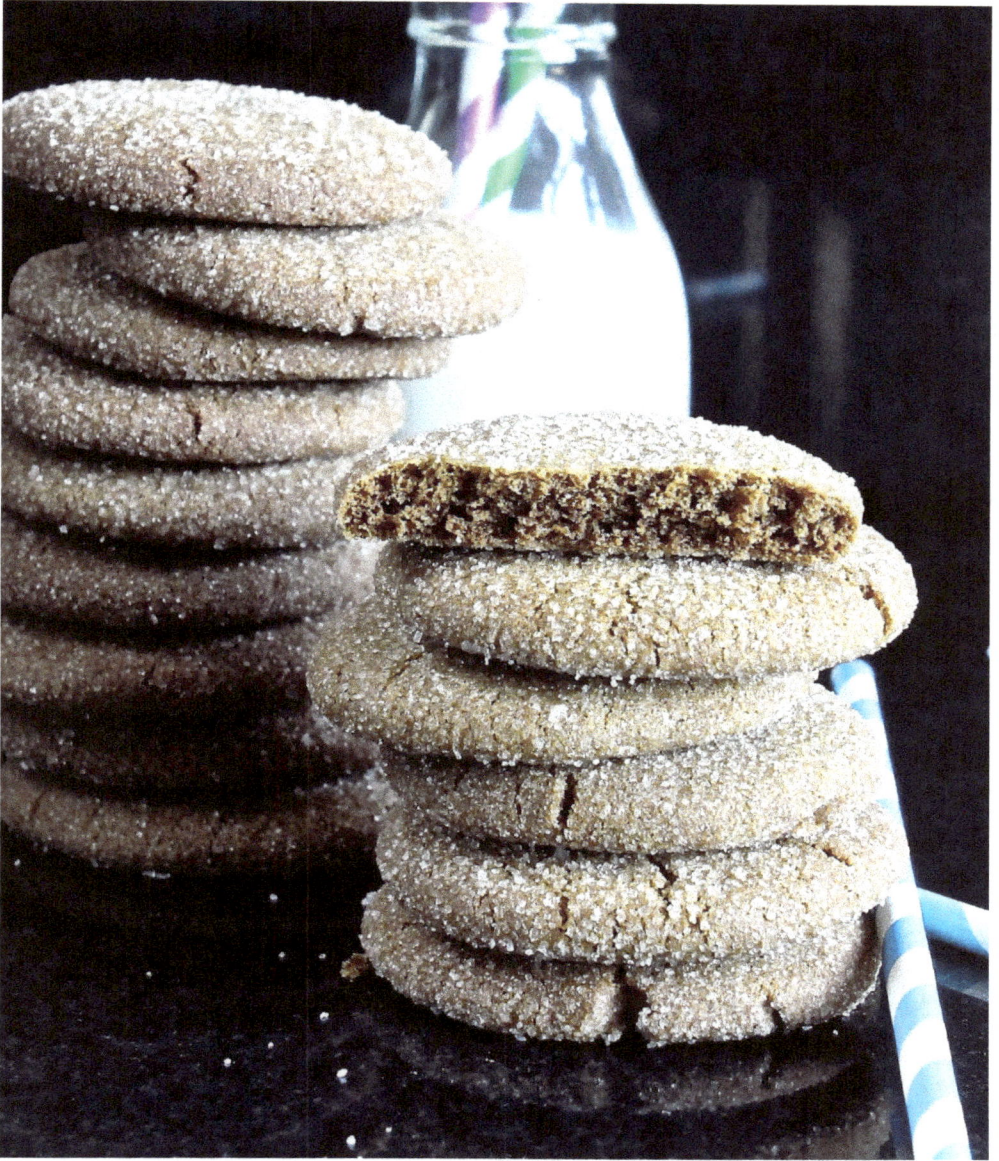

Low Cholesterol-Low Calorie Blueberry Muffin

Time To Prepare: ten minutes

Time to Cook: twenty-five minutes

Yield: Servings 12

Ingredients:

- ½ cup skim milk or non-fat milk
- ½ cup white sugar
- 1 and ½ cup of flour, all-purpose
- 1 cup blueberries, fresh
- 1 egg white
- 1 tablespoon coconut oil
- 2 tablespoons melted margarine
- 2 teaspoons baking powder
- Pinch of salt

Directions:

1. Set the oven to 205C.
2. Grease a 12-cup muffin pan using oil.
3. In a small container, put the blueberries. Put in ¼ cup of the flour and mix it together. Set aside.

4. In another container, whisk the egg white and the coconut oil. Put in the melted margarine.

5. In a different container, mix all together the dry ingredients and sift. Sift again over the egg white mixture. Mix to moisten the flour. The flour should look lumpy, so do not overmix.

6. Fold in the blueberries. Separate the blueberries, so that each scoop will have blueberries. Scoop the mixture into the muffin pans. Fill only up to two-thirds of the pan.

7. Bake for about twenty-five minutes or until the muffin turns golden brown.

Nutritional Info: ‖ Calories: 114 kcal ‖ Protein: 2.66 g ‖ Fat: 5.34 g ‖ Carbohydrates: 14.25 g

Mandarin Cottage Cheese

Time To Prepare: five minutes

Time to Cook: 0 minutes

Yield: Servings 1

Ingredients:

- ½ cup canned mandarin oranges
- ½ cup low-fat cottage cheese
- 1 ½ tablespoons slivered almonds

Directions:

1. Put the cottage cheese in a container.
2. Drain the mandarin oranges, put them atop the cottage cheese, and drizzle with almonds.

Nutritional Info: ‖ Calories: 360 kcal ‖ Protein: 26.24 g ‖ Fat: 21.37 g ‖ Carbohydrates: 15.22 g

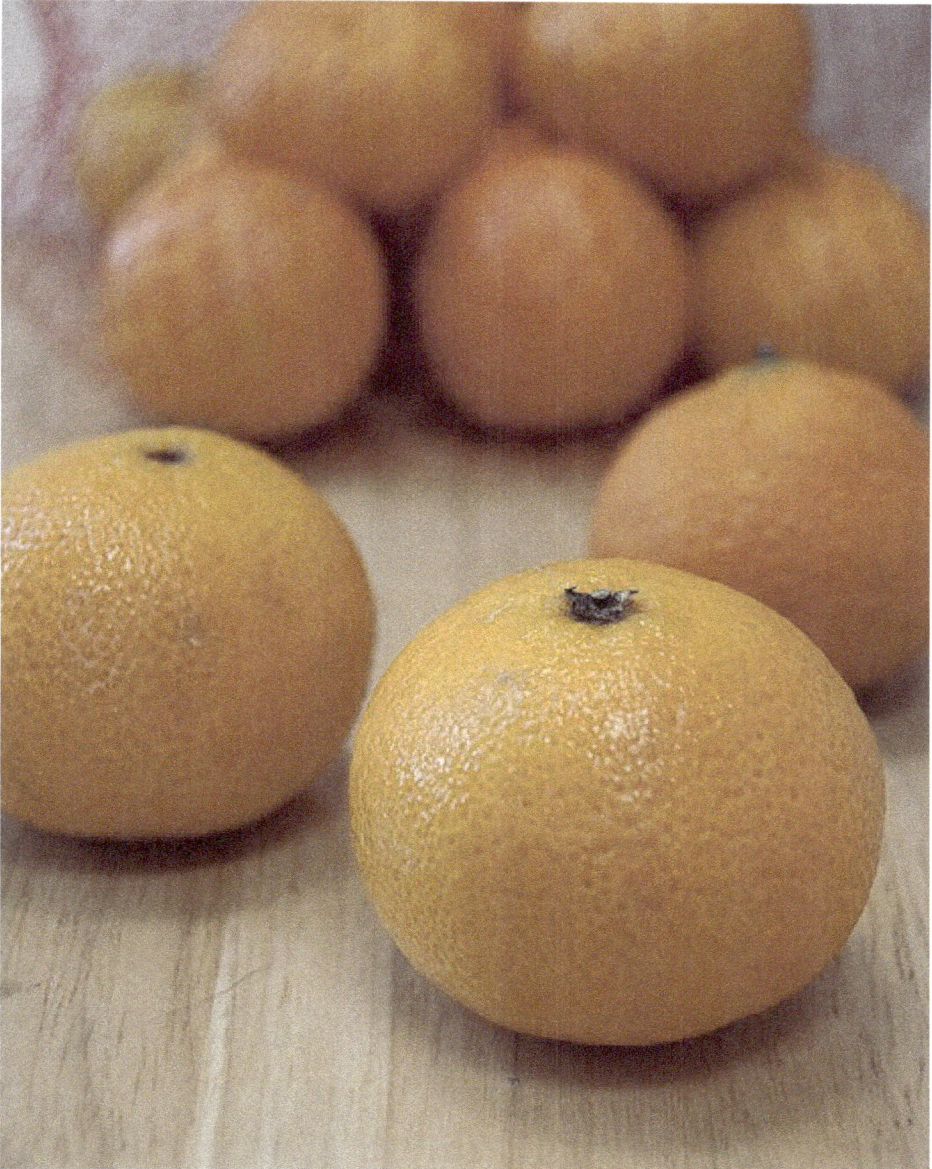

Mini Pepper Nachos

Time To Prepare: five minutes

Time to Cook: ten minutes

Yield: Servings 8

Ingredients:

- .25 tsp. Red pepper flakes
- .5 cup Tomato, chopped
- .5 tsp. Oregano
- 1 tbsp. Chili powder
- 1 tsp. Cumin, ground
- 1 tsp. Garlic powder
- 1 tsp. Paprika
- 16 oz. Ground beef
- 16 oz. Mini peppers, seeded, halved
- 5 tsp. Pepper
- 5 tsp. Salt
- cup Cheddar cheese, shredded

Directions:

1. Mix seasonings together in a container.
2. On moderate heat, brown the meat, be sure all the clumps are broken up.

3. Stir in the spices and continue to sauté until the seasoning has gone through all of the meat.

4. Heat the oven to 400F.

5. Put the peppers in a single line. They can touch.

6. Coat with the beef mix.

7. Drizzle with cheese.

8. Bake for minimum ten minutes or until cheese has melted.

9. Pull out of the oven and top with the toppings.

Nutritional Info: ‖ Calories: 240 kcal ‖ Protein: 11.01 g ‖ Fat: 18.2 g ‖ Carbohydrates: 9.49 g

Mushroom Chips

Time To Prepare: ten minutes

Time to Cook: 45-60 minutes

Yield: Servings 2-4

Ingredients:

- 16 ounces of king oyster mushrooms
- 2 tablespoons ghee
- Kosher salt and ground pepper to taste

Directions:

1. Set the oven to 300F, then line two cookie sheets using parchment paper.
2. Cut every mushroom in half along the length, then cut with a mandolin into 1/8 inch slices or strips. Put them on cookie sheets with some room in between. Melt the ghee and brush it over the mushrooms, then flavor with the salt and pepper.
3. Bake for minimum 45 minutes to an hour, until they are completely crunchy. Store in airtight containers.

Nutritional Info: ‖ Calories: 62 kcal ‖ Protein: 5.58 g ‖ Fat: 2 g ‖ Carbohydrates: 7.97 g

SOUPS AND STEWS

Lemon Chicken Soup

Time To Prepare: ten minutes
Time to Cook: 4 hours
Yield: Servings 4

Ingredients:

- ¼ cup freshly squeezed lemon juice
- 1 yellow onion, chopped
- 2 boneless, skinless chicken breasts
- 2 cloves garlic, chopped
- 2 tablespoons chives, chopped
- 6 cups chicken broth
- Salt & pepper, to taste

Directions:

1. Put in all the ingredients to a slow cooker and cook on high for 4 hours.
2. Once cooked, shred the chicken and stir back into the soup.

Nutritional Info: Calories: 171 ‖ Carbohydrates: 6g ‖ Fiber: 1g Net ‖ Carbohydrates: 5g ‖ Fat: 6g ‖ Protein: 22g

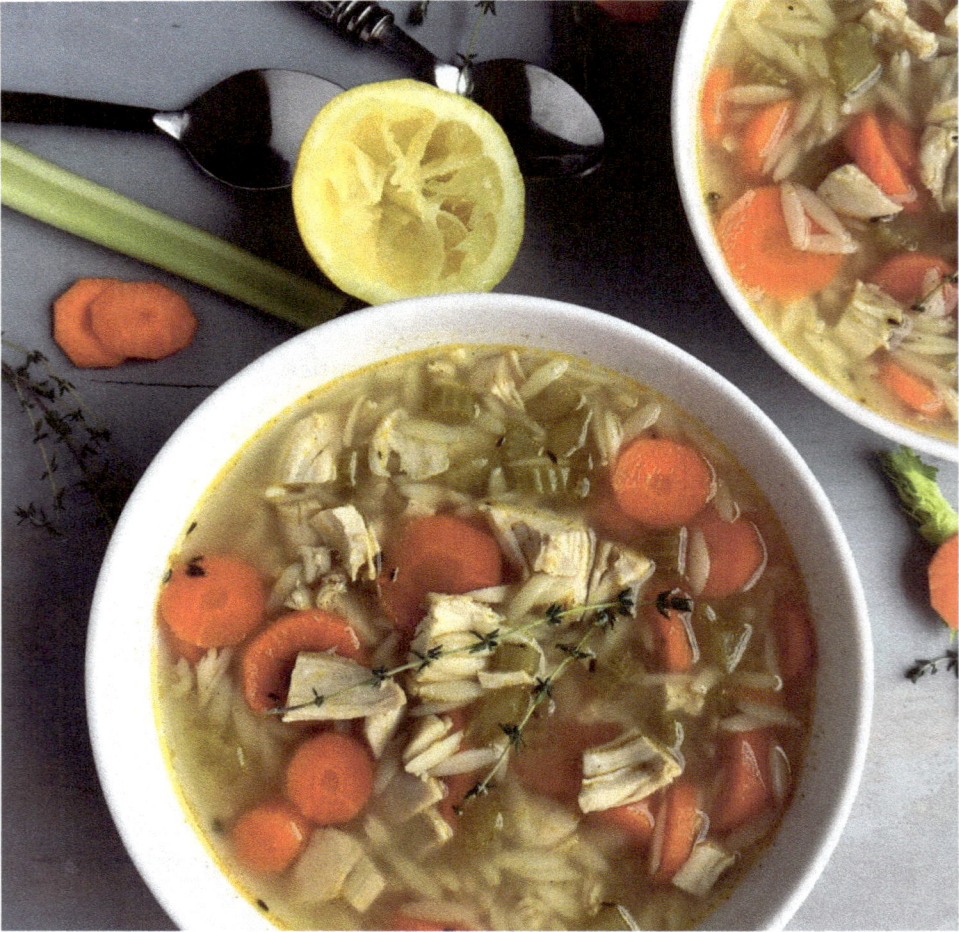

Mediterranean Stew

Time To Prepare: ten minutes

Time to Cook: fifteen minutes

Yield: Servings 4

Ingredients:

- 1 (19-ounce) can cannellini beans, drained and washed
- 1 (fifteen½-ounce) can chickpeas, drained and washed
- 1 cup Basic Vegetable Stock or low-sodium canned vegetable stock
- 1 teaspoon dried oregano
- 1 teaspoon red pepper, crushed or to taste
- 1½ cups artichoke hearts, quartered
- 2 cups roasted tomatoes
- 3 cloves garlic, crushed and minced
- 3 tablespoons olive oil
- 4 tablespoons grated Parmesan cheese
- Chopped Italian parsley, for decoration
- Chopped sun-dried tomatoes, for decoration
- Crumbled feta cheese, for decoration
- Fresh oregano leaves, for decoration
- Freshly ground black pepper, to taste

- Garlic-seasoned croutons, for decoration
- Salt, to taste

Directions:

1. Warm the olive oil in a huge deep cooking pan on moderate heat and sauté the garlic for two to three minutes or until golden.
2. Lower the heat to moderate-low. Mix in the chickpeas, cannellini beans, roasted tomatoes, artichoke hearts, stock, Parmesan cheese, crushed red pepper, oregano, salt, and pepper. Cook and stir for approximately ten minutes. Serve in separate bowls, garnishing as you wish.

Nutritional Info: Calories: 445 ‖ Fat: 16 g ‖ Protein: 18 g ‖ Sodium: 530 mg ‖ Fiber: 12 g ‖ Carbohydrates: 61 g

Minestrone Soup with Quinoa

Time To Prepare: ten minutes

Time to Cook: twenty minutes

Yield: Servings 6

Ingredients:

- ½ cup quinoa, washed well
- ½ red bell pepper, diced
- ½ teaspoon salt
- 1 (14 oz.) can cannellini beans, drained and washed well
- 1 (14 oz.) can diced tomatoes with its juice
- 1 bay leaf
- 1 cup packed kale, stemmed and meticulously washed
- 1 medium white onion, diced
- 1 small zucchini, diced
- 1 tablespoon freshly squeezed lemon juice
- 1 tablespoon ghee
- 2 carrots, chopped
- 2 celery stalks, diced
- 2 garlic cloves, minced
- 2 teaspoons dried rosemary
- 2 teaspoons dried thyme

- 5 cups vegetable broth
- Freshly ground black pepper

Directions:

1. In a huge soup pot on moderate heat, put in the ghee, garlic, onion, carrots, and celery, and sauté for about three minutes.
2. Put in the zucchini and red bell pepper, and sauté for a couple of minutes.
3. Mix in the broth, tomatoes, beans, kale, quinoa, lemon juice, rosemary, thyme, bay leaf, and salt, and flavor with black pepper. Put it to a simmer, reduce the heat temperature, cover, and cook for fifteen minutes, or until the quinoa is cooked. Take away the bay leaf and discard it. Serve hot.

Nutritional Info: Calories: 319 ‖ Total Fat: 5g ‖ Saturated Fat: 2g ‖ Cholesterol: 0mg ‖ Carbohydrates: 42g ‖ Fiber: 9g ‖ Protein: 18g

Moong Daal

Time To Prepare: fifteen minutes

Time to Cook: thirty minutes

Yield: Servings 6

Ingredients:

- ½ Cup Tomatoes (Diced)
- ½ Dried Red Chili Pepper
- ½ Teaspoon Ginger Root (Grated)
- ½ Teaspoon Ground Turmeric
- 1 Pinch Asafoetida
- 1 Teaspoon Cumin Seed
- 1 Teaspoon Jalapeno (Diced)
- 1/4 Cup Cilantro (Chopped)
- 2 Cloves Garlic (Chopped)
- 2 Teaspoons Vegetable Oil
- 2½ Cups Moong Dal (Rinsed)
- 2½ Cups Water
- 3 Teaspoons Lemon Juice
- Salt

Directions:

1. Soak daal for thirty minutes before boiling in water with salt until thick.
2. Put in ginger, jalapeno, tomato, lemon juice, and turmeric.
3. Heat cumin seed and red Chile pepper in a pan before you put in asafoetida powder and garlic.
4. Combine with split peas and serve with cilantro.

Nutritional Info: Calories: 330 kcal ‖ Carbohydrates: 57 g ‖ Fat: 3 g ‖ Protein: 21 g

Mushroom And Thyme Soup

Time To Prepare: five minutes

Time to Cook: twenty minutes

Yield: Servings 4

Ingredients:

- ¼ cup butter
- 12 ounces (340 g) wild mushrooms, chopped
- 2 garlic cloves, minced
- 2 teaspoons thyme leaves
- 4 cups vegetable broth
- 5 ounces (142 g) crème fraiche
- From the cupboard:
- Salt and freshly ground black pepper, to taste

Directions:

1. Place the butter in a deep cooking pan and melt on moderate heat.
2. Put in the minced garlic and cook for a minutes or until aromatic.
3. Put in the chopped mushrooms, and drizzle with salt and black pepper. Stir to blend and cook for about ten minutes or until the mushrooms are soft.

4. Put in the vegetable broth and bring the soup to its boiling point. Stir continuously. Reduce the heat and simmer the soup for about ten minutes or until it becomes slightly thick.
5. Pour the soup in a blender, and pulse until smooth, then fold in the crème fraiche.
6. Move the soup in a big container and top with thyme leaves before you serve.

Nutritional Info: calories: 282 ‖ total fat: 25.1g ‖ net carbs: 6.3g ‖ protein: 7.8g

Onion, Kale and White Bean Soup

Time To Prepare: fifteen minutes

Time to Cook: twenty-five minutes

Yield: Servings 4

Ingredients:

- ⅛ Teaspoon red pepper flakes (not necessary)
- ¼ cup extra-virgin olive oil
- ¼ teaspoon freshly ground black pepper
- 1 (fifteen½-ounce) can white beans, drained and washed
- 1 big onion, thinly cut
- 1 teaspoon finely chopped fresh rosemary
- 1 teaspoon salt
- 2 garlic cloves, thinly cut
- 3 cups stemmed kale leaves cut into ½-inch pieces
- 4 cups vegetable broth

Directions:

1. In a large pot, heat the oil on high heat.
2. Lower the heat to moderate, and put in the onion, garlic, salt, pepper, and red pepper flakes (if using).

Sauté until the onion is golden, approximately ten minutes.

3. Put in the kale, and sauté until wilted, one to two minutes.

4. Pour the broth then bring to its boiling point.

5. Lower the heat to simmer, and cook until the kale is tender about five minutes.

6. Put in the beans and rosemary. Cook until the beans are warmed through minimum two to three minutes before you serve.

Nutritional Info: Calories: 285 ‖ Total Fat: 15g ‖ Total Carbohydrates: 28g ‖ Sugar: 3g ‖ Fiber: 9g ‖ Protein: 13g ‖ Sodium: 1368mg

Pork Stew

Time To Prepare: five minutes
Time to Cook: 8 hours
Yield: Servings 6

Ingredients:

- 1 onion, finely chopped
- 1 teaspoon dried mixed spices (homemade or store-bought)
- 2 pounds (907 g) pork loin, cut into cubes
- 2 tablespoons olive oil
- 3 cups chicken stock
- 4 garlic cloves, crushed
- From the cupboard:
- Salt and freshly ground black pepper, to taste

Directions:

1. Grease the insert of the slow cooker with olive oil.
2. Combine the pork, chicken stock, onion, dried mixed spices, garlic, salt, and black pepper in the slow cooker.
3. Place the slow cooker lid on and cook on LOW for eight hours.
4. Ladle the stew in a big container and serve warm.

Nutritional Info: calories: 381 ‖ total fat: 18.3g ‖ carbs: 9.2g ‖ protein: 42.3g

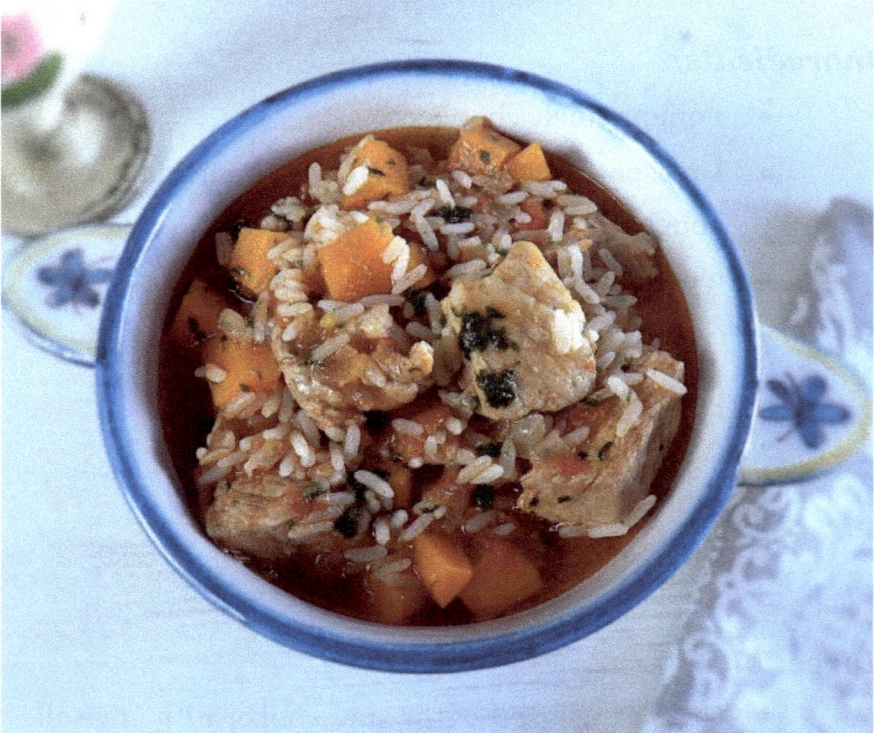

Pumpkin And Sausage Soup

Time To Prepare: five minutes

Time to Cook: 33 minutes

Yield: Servings 4

Ingredients:

- ½ cup heavy whipping cream
- ½ cup pumpkin puree
- ½ teaspoon dried sage
- ½ teaspoon ground dried thyme
- ½ teaspoon red chili pepper flakes (not necessary)
- 1 garlic clove, minced
- 1 moderate-sized red onion, minced
- 1 pinch salt
- 1 small red bell pepper, diced
- 2 cups chicken broth
- 2 tablespoons butter, melted
- pounds (680 g) fresh sausage

Directions:

1. Sauté the sausage in a nonstick frying pan on moderate to high heat for a minutes, then put in the onion and bell pepper. Continue sautéing for about six

minutes until the sausage is mildly browned and the onion is translucent.

2. Fold in the chili pepper flakes, thyme, sage, minced garlic, and salt, then put in the pumpkin puree, chicken broth, and heavy whipping cream.

3. Reduce the heat and bring them to a simmer using low heat for fifteen minutes or until it becomes thick.

4. Pour the cooked soup into a big serving container and put in the butter. Stir to mix thoroughly before you serve.

Nutritional Info: calories: 777 ‖ total fat: 70g ‖ net carbs: 7g ‖ fiber: 2g ‖ protein: 27g

Pumpkin, Coconut & Sage Soup

Time To Prepare: fifteen minutes

Time to Cook: thirty minutes

Yield: Servings 6

Ingredients:

- 1 cup canned pumpkin
- 1 cup full-fat coconut milk
- 1 teaspoon freshly chopped sage
- 2 cloves garlic, chopped
- 6 cups vegetable broth
- Pinch of salt & pepper, to taste

Directions:

1. Put in all the ingredients minus the coconut milk to a stockpot on moderate heat and bring to its boiling point. Reduce to a simmer and cook for half an hour
2. Put in the coconut milk and stir.

Nutritional Info: Calories: 146 ‖ Carbohydrates: 7g ‖ Fiber: 2g Net ‖ Carbohydrates: 5g ‖ Fat: 11g ‖ Protein: 6g

DESSERTS

Mediterranean Rolled Baklava With Walnuts

Time To Prepare: twenty minutes

Time to Cook: forty minutes

Yield: Servings 12

Ingredients:

- 1 cup Cream of wheat or plain breadcrumbs
- 1 Lemon zest
- 1 medium Lemon
- 1/3 cup Milk
- 2 cups Walnuts
- 3 cups Granulated sugar
- 3 cups Water
- 3 sticks Melted Unsalted butter
- 3 tbsp. Sugar
- 8 sheets Thawed phyllo dough
- Syrup:

Directions:

1. Mix 3 cups of sugar, 3 cups of water and lemon slices in a pan and leave to boil

2. Reduce the heat, then allow it to simmer until the sugar completely dissolves. It should take fifteen minutes. You should have a nice smooth syrup now. Now allow to cool for a bit.

3. Cut the walnuts in a blender into bits using short pulses.

4. Pour the walnuts in a container together with the cream of wheat, lemon zest and 4 tablespoons of sugar.

5. Mix in milk and save for later.

6. Now, preheat the oven to 375°F.

7. Spread out the phyllo dough and fit it into a baking pan. Trim off the edges that do not fit with scissors. Cover the rest of the phyllo sheets while you work so they do not dry out.

8. Put a sheet on a clean flat surface and glaze with melted butter. Do this for all the sheets until it's finished.

9. Position the walnut mixture on one side of the sheets and roll them up like you're trying to make a sausage. Do this for all the sheets and walnuts.

10. Position the walnut rolls on an ungreased baking pan and glaze with the leftover butter.

11. Bake for approximately 45 minutes. It's ready when it looks golden.

12. Turn off the oven then pull out the baking pan. Sprinkle syrup over the baklava, ensuring the syrup gets everywhere.

13. Bring back the baking pan into the oven then let sit for five minutes.

14. Remove from the oven and allow to cool for a few hours. Cut the rolls into small amounts before you serve.

Nutritional Info: ‖ Calories: 488 kcal ‖ Protein: 4.49 g ‖ Fat: 36.89 g ‖ Carbohydrates: 38.21 g

Mint Chocolate Chip Ice-cream

Time To Prepare: five minutes

Time to Cook: 0 minutes

Yield: Servings 2

Ingredients:

- ½ cup Raw cashews or coconut cream, optional.
- 1/8 tsp. Pure peppermint extract
- 2 Frozen overripe bananas
- 3 tbsp. Chocolate chips or sugar-free chocolate chips
- Pinch Salt
- Pinch Spirulina or any natural food coloring, optional.

Directions:

1. Mint or imitation peppermint won't be a substitute for this. Use pure peppermint extract and pour in slowly.
2. Peel and chop the bananas first. Put the slices in a Ziplock bag then freeze.
3. For the ice cream, put all the ingredients in a blender and pulse. You can skip the chocolate chips and just put in them after blending.
4. Serve the moment it's ready or freeze until it's firm enough, then serve!

Nutritional Info: ‖ Calories: 250 kcal ‖ Protein: 6.13 g ‖ Fat: 24.37 g ‖ Carbohydrates: 7.72 g

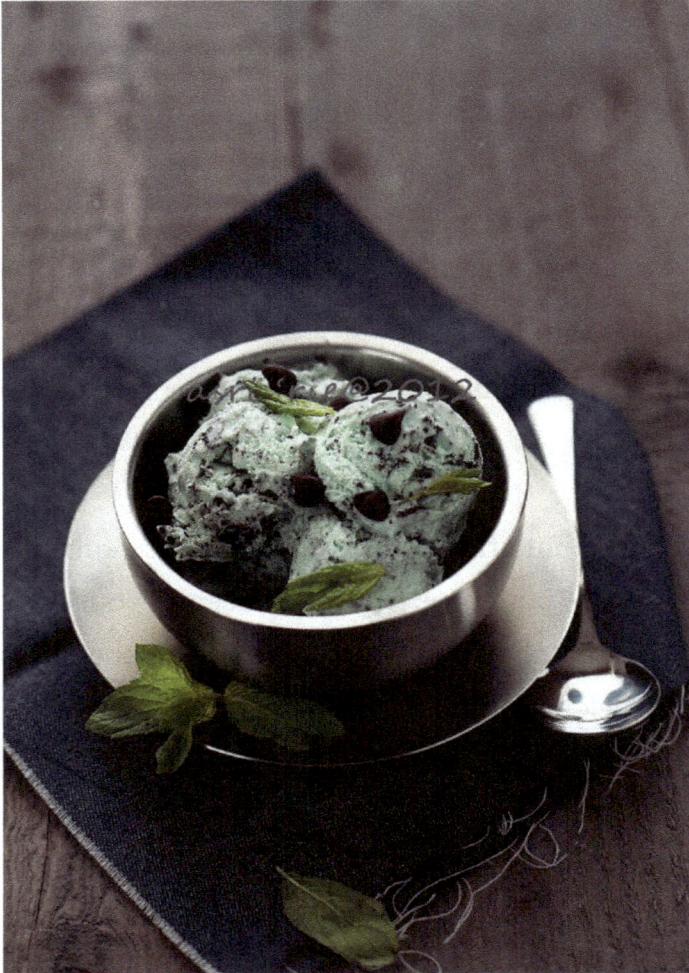

No-Bake Carrot Cake Bites

Time To Prepare: fifteen minutes

Time to Cook: 0 minutes

Yield: Servings 6

Ingredients:

- ½ teaspoon of ground ginger
- ¾ cup of shredded coconut
- 1 and a ½ cups of carrots
- 1 cup of pitted Medjool dates
- 1 cup of walnuts
- 1 tablespoon of pure maple syrup
- 1 teaspoon of cinnamon

Directions:

1. Put all together the ingredients into a high-speed blender or food processor, and blend until the mixture comes together, putting in a teaspoon of water at a time if required.
2. Take the carrot mixture and press down into a cupcake tin, and place in your fridge until firm.
3. Pop the carrot cakes out of the muffin tin, and enjoy!

Nutritional Info: ‖ Total Carbohydrates: 32g ‖ Fiber: 5g ‖ Net Carbohydrates: ‖ Protein: 3g ‖ Total Fat: 12g ‖ Calories: 231

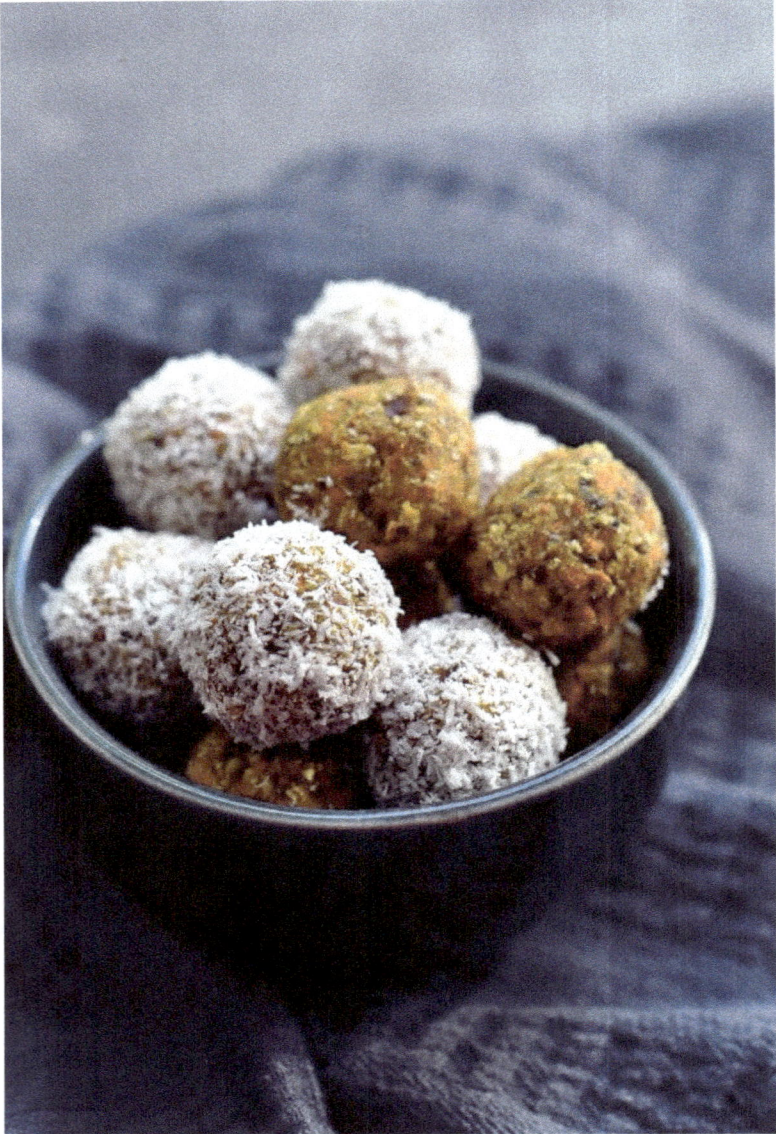

No-Bake Cheesecake

Time To Prepare: twenty minutes

Time to Cook: 0 minutes

Yield: Servings 12

Ingredients:

For Crust:

- 1 cup of dates (pitted and chopped)
- 1 cup of raw almonds
- two to three tablespoons of unsweetened coconut, shredded

For Filling:

- ½ cup of coconut oil, melted
- ¾ cup of fresh lemon juice
- ¾ cup of raw honey
- 1 teaspoon of organic vanilla extract
- 10 drops of liquid stevia
- 2 tablespoons of fresh lemon rind, grated finely
- 3½ cups of cashews, soaked overnight
- A thinly cut lemon
- Salt

Directions:

1. Put together the dates, almonds, and coconut in a blender and pulse.
2. Move the puree a greased springform pan.
3. Smooth the outer lining of the crust using a spatula.
4. Put cashews and oil in a food processor and pulse.
5. Put in the rest of the ingredients except for lemon slices and pulse until it turns creamy and smooth.
6. Put the combination over the crust uniformly.
7. Smooth the counter of filling using the corner of a spatula.
8. Place in your fridge for one hour.
9. Take it off from the fridge and decorate with lemon slices.
10. Chop it into desired sized slices before you serve.

Nutritional Info: ‖ Calories: 468 ‖ Fat: 32g ‖ Carbohydrates: 6.6g ‖ Sugar: 44.1g ‖ Protein: 8.4g ‖ Sodium: 23mg

Paleo Raspberry Cream Pie

Time To Prepare: twenty minutes

Time to Cook: 0 minutes

Yield: Servings 12

Ingredients:
For the crust:
- ½ cup Unsweetened shredded coconut
- 1 ½ tbsp. Maple syrup
- 1 cup Roasted or salted cashews
- 1 tsp. Vanilla extract
- Pinch Salt

Raspberry filling:
- ¼ cup & 2 tsp. Fresh lemon juice
- ¼ cup Coconut cream from the top solid part of a can of coconut milk that has been placed in the fridge overnight
- ½ cup & 1 tbsp. Maple syrup
- ¾ cup Unrefined coconut oil
- 1 ½ cup Roasted or salted cashews
- 2 tsp. Vanilla extract
- 3 cups Fresh raspberries
- Pinch Salt

Directions:

1. Prepare 12 muffin pans, line them with muffin liners, and set them aside.

2. Make the crust. Set a pan on moderate heat and the coconut and stir until it's completely toasted. Stay by the pan because coconuts tend to burn very easily.

3. Move the toasted coconuts to a container and leave to cool for five minutes or so. Honestly, this toasting step isn't particularly necessary, but I feel it adds amazing flavor to the crust.

4. To make the crust, put all the ingredients in a blender and pulse at the lowest speed until the mix gets all clumpy. Also, do not pulse for too long, or you might end up with a paste. To know if it's ready, put a small amount of the mixture on your fingers and pinch. If it gets clumpy, you're on track, if not, put in a little water and pulse at the lowest speed for further minutes.

5. Scoop the mix into the lined tins using your fingers to pack the mix firmly inside the pan.

6. Place the pans to place in your fridge while you get to make the filling.

7. In a tiny pot set using low heat, mix in all the ingredients until the oil and coconut cream melts completely. Clean the blender using a paper towel and pour in the filling.

8. Pulse at high-speed for like 60 seconds or until it's super smooth. The only clumps we can forgive are the raspberry seeds.

9. Sprinkle a quarter of the filling over the top of each crust. There must be extra filling; you can store and use that in a different dish.

10. Put the coated muffins in your refrigerator to cool. This will take a few hours, like 6 hours, so if you do not have time for that, put it in the freezer.

11. To serve, allow them to defrost for 80 minutes or until obviously creamy.

Nutritional Info: ‖ Calories: 565 kcal ‖ Protein: 7.74 g ‖ Fat: 43.72 g ‖ Carbohydrates: 42.72 g

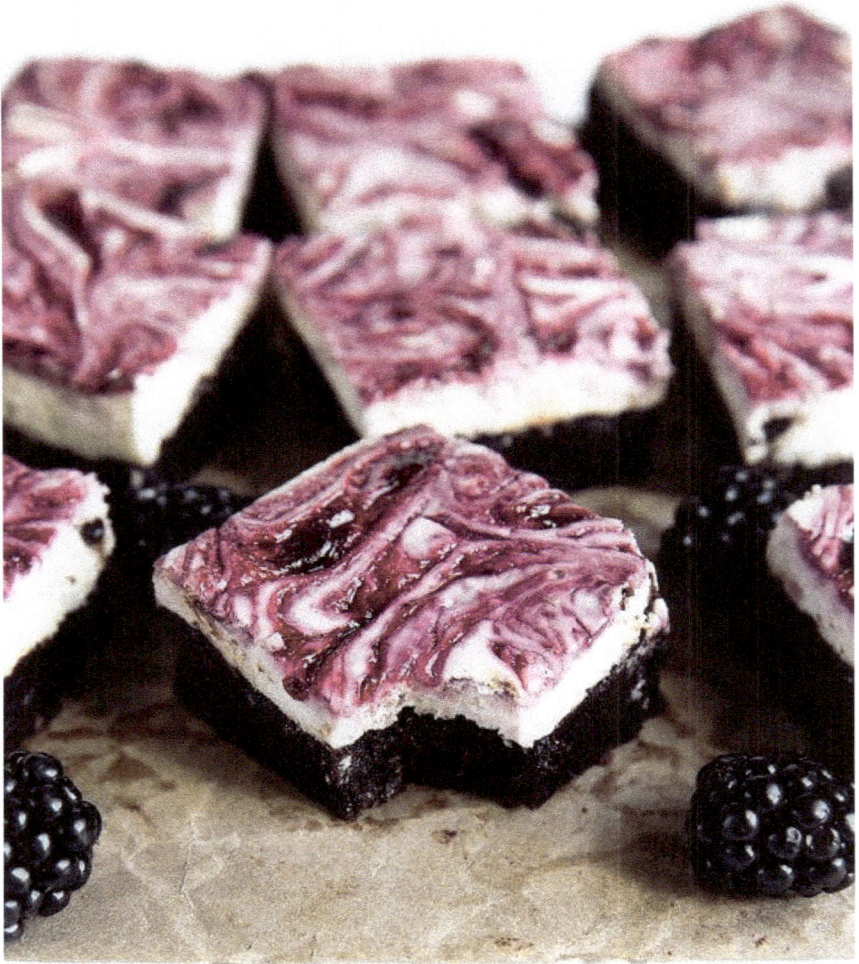

Peanut Butter Balls

Time To Prepare: twenty minutes
Time to Cook: thirty minutes
Yield: Servings 5

Ingredients:

- 1 Tsp. Vanilla Extract
- 2 Tbsp. Peanut Oil.
- 200g Powdered Sugar
- 250g Chocolate
- 250g Creamy Peanut Butter
- 90g Melted Butter

Direction:

1. Mix everything apart from the oil and chocolates to make a batter
2. Place in your fridge the batter for about forty-five minutes.
3. Make small balls with the batter using and put them on a parchment paper. Place in your fridge for one more hour.
4. Melt some dark chocolate. Place the peanut balls into the chocolate and place in your fridge for about twenty minutes.

5. Serve with strawberry.

Nutritional Info: ‖ Calories: 340 kcal ‖ Carbohydrates: 32 g ‖ Fat: 21 g ‖ Protein: 1.4 g.

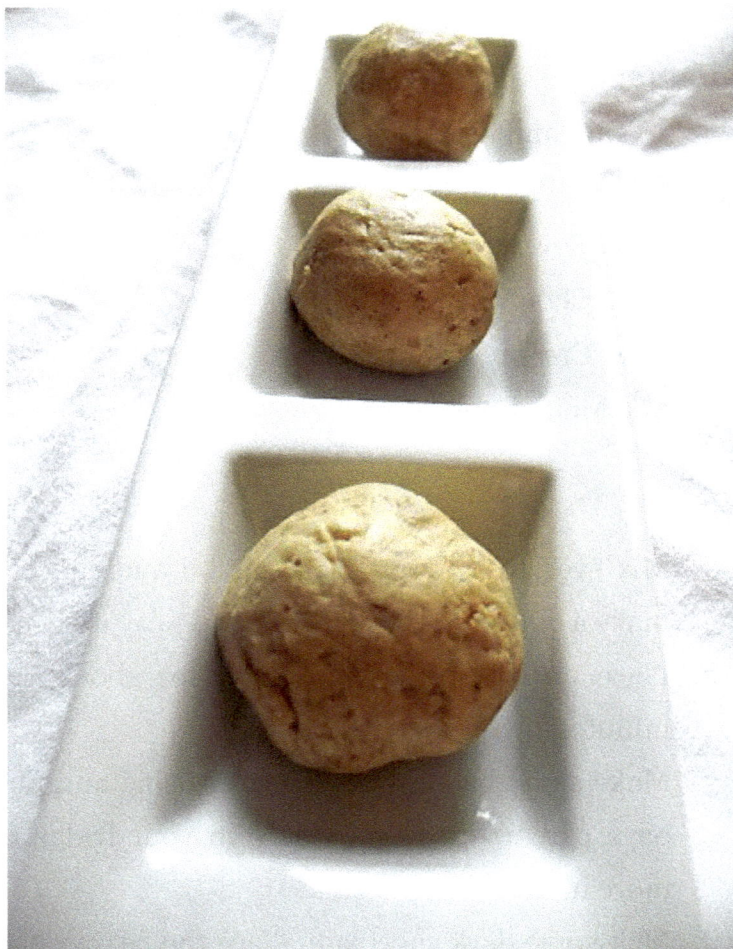

Peanut Butter Cookies

Time To Prepare: fifteen Minutes

Time to Cook: 0 Minute

Yield: Servings 9

Ingredients:

- ½ a cup of peanut butter (creamy and unsalted)
- 1 and a ¼ teaspoon of vanilla extract
- 1 cup of pitted Medjool dates
- 1 cup of raw almonds
- Sea salt as required

Directions:

1. Take a food processor and put in almonds, peanut butter, vanilla, dates and blend the whole mixture until a dough-like texture comes (should take a few minutes)
2. If you desire, put in some more peanut butter to make the dough sticker.
3. Form balls using the dough and press down using a fork to create a criss-cross pattern
4. Drizzle salt liberally
5. Serve instantly.

Nutritional Info: ‖ Calories: 350 Cal ‖ Fat: 17 g ‖ Carbohydrates: 27 g ‖ Protein: 18 g

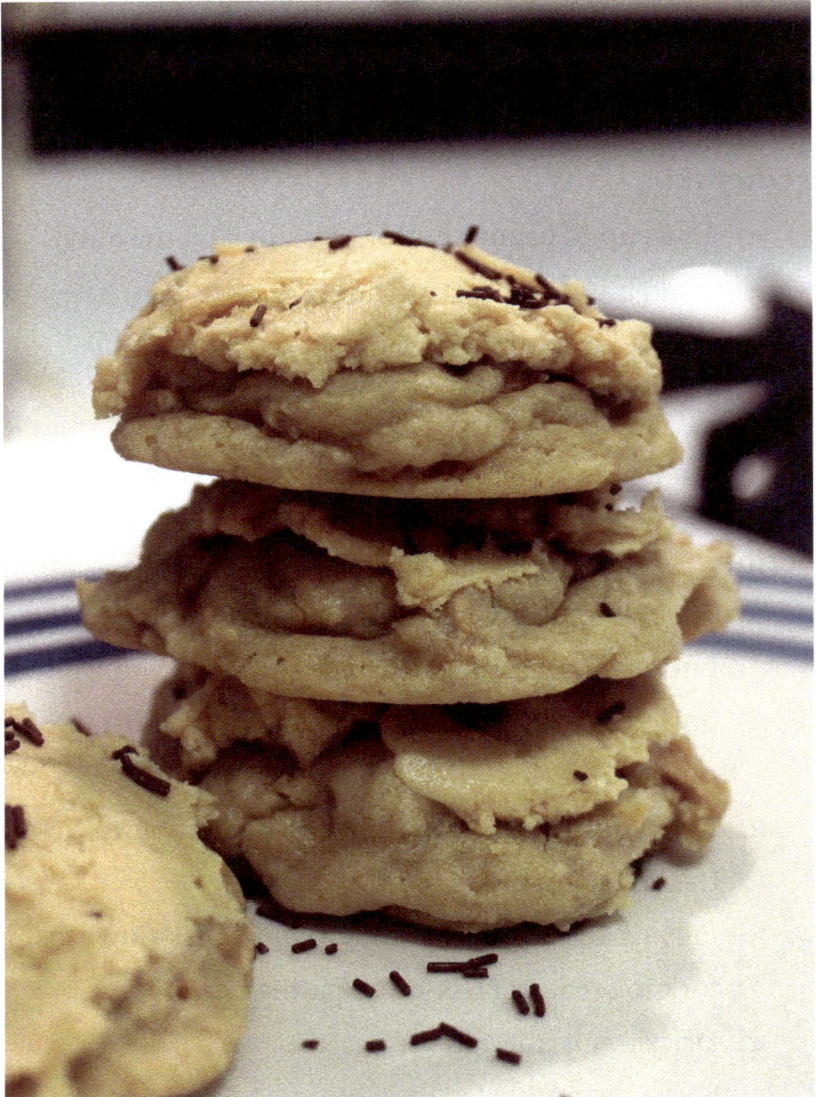

Pineapple Cake

Time To Prepare: fifteen minutes

Time to Cook: 50 minutes

Yield: Servings 8

Ingredients:

- ½ tsp. Baking powder
- 1 tbsp. Almond flour
- 1 tsp. Vanilla extract
- 2 slices Fresh pineapples
- 2 Whole medium eggs
- 3 tbsp. Melted coconut oil
- 5 tbsp. Raw honey
- fifteen pcs. Frozen sweet cherries

Directions:

1. Preheat your oven to 350°F.
2. Take away the skin and core of the pineapples. Set aside.
3. Sprinkle 1½ tablespoons of raw honey in a round cake tin.
4. Layer the pineapple rings and sweet cherries on the honey in a decorative fashion.

5. Bring the cake tin in your oven then bake for fifteen minutes.

6. While all that is going on, mix in the almond and baking powder.

7. In a different container, mix the eggs and leftover honey. Sprinkle in coconut oil and stir.

8. Now put in the almond mix to the egg mix and stir meticulously.

9. Take out the cake tin and sprinkle batter over the top of the partly baked pineapple rings and use a spatula to spread it uniformly.

10. Place the cake tin back in your oven and bake for an additional thirty-five minutes.

11. When it's all set, take it out of the oven and leave it to sit for about ten minutes before place it to a plate.

12. Serve with extra cherries if you prefer.

Nutritional Info: ‖ Calories: 120 kcal ‖ Protein: 2.3 g ‖ Fat: 6.99 g ‖ Carbohydrates: 12.98 g

Pineapple Pie

Time To Prepare: fifteen minutes
Time to Cook: 50 minutes
Yield: Servings 8

Ingredients:

- ½-tsp baking powder
- 1-cup almond flour
- 1-tsp pure vanilla extract
- 2-pcs eggs
- 2-pcs fresh pineapple, peeled, cored, and cut into rings
- 3-Tbsps liquid coconut oil
- 5-Tbsps raw honey (divided)
- fifteen-pcs sweet cherries, fresh or frozen

Directions:

1. Preheat the oven to 350 °F.
2. Pour 1½-tablespoon of the honey in a round baking tin. Position the cherries and pineapple rings on the bed of honey in a decorative pattern. Put the pan in your oven, then bake for minimum fifteen minutes.
3. Meanwhile, mix in all the rest of the ingredients in a mixing container. Mix thoroughly until forming the mixture into dough. Set aside.

4. Take the pan out from the oven. Push down the batter over the pineapple rings, smoothing it at the top.

5. Return the pan in your oven, and bake further for a little more than half an hour.

Nutritional Info: ‖ Calories: 213 ‖ Fat: 7.1g ‖ Protein: 15.9g ‖ Sodium: 39.2mg ‖ Total Carbohydrates: 23.7g ‖ Fiber: 2.4g ‖ Net Carbohydrates: 21.3g

Pistachioed Panna-Cotta Cocoa

Time To Prepare: eighteen minutes
Time to Cook: two minutes
Yield: Servings 6

Ingredients:

- 12-oz. dark chocolate
- 1-Tbsp coconut oil
- 3-pcs big bananas, cut into thirds
- Cocoa nibs, chopped
- Salted pistachios, chopped
- Spiced or smoked almonds, chopped

Directions:

1. Coat a baking pan using parchment paper.
2. Melt the dark chocolate with oil in your microwave. Set aside.
3. Pierce a Popsicle stick midway into one end of each banana.
4. Immerse each banana into the melted chocolate. Put dipped bananas into the baking sheet. Drizzle liberally with the cocoa nibs, almonds, and pistachios. Put the sheet in your freezer to harden and set.

Nutritional Info: ‖ Calories: 454 ‖ Fat: 15.1g ‖ Protein: 22.7g ‖ Sodium: 91mg ‖ Total Carbohydrates: 61.6g ‖ Fiber: 4.9g ‖ Net Carbohydrates: 56.7g

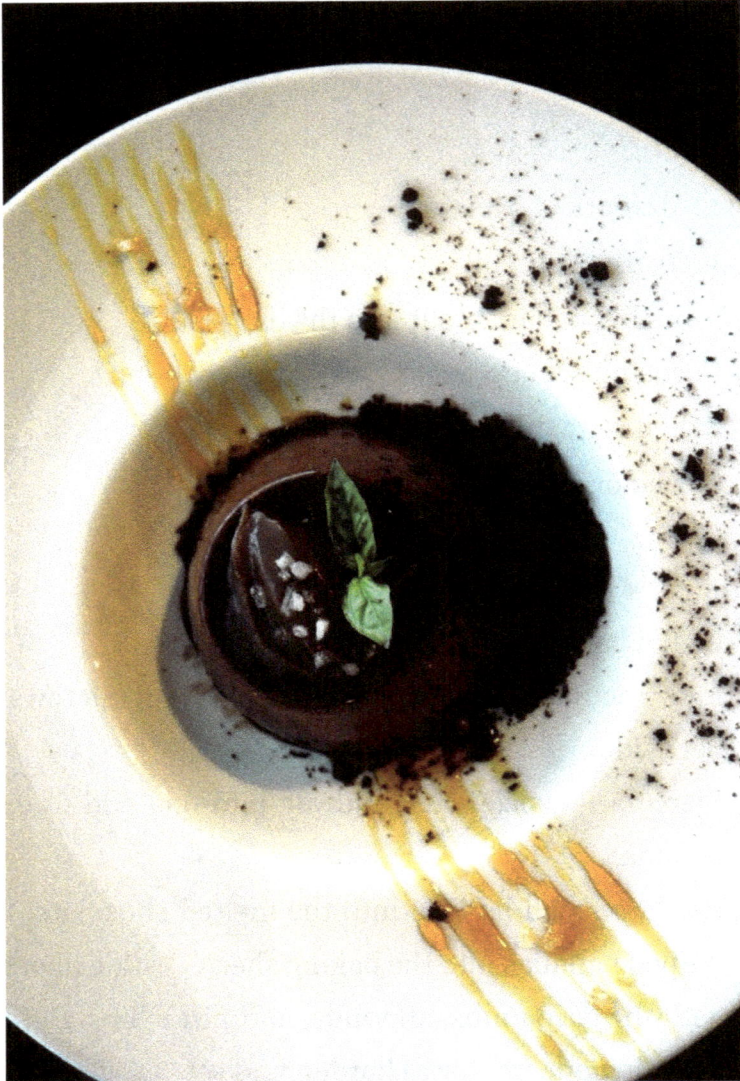

www.ingramcontent.com/pod-product-compliance
Lightning Source LLC
Chambersburg PA
CBHW071108030426
42336CB00013BA/1998